PREVENTIVE MEDICINE

NEVER GET SICK

Complete Guide to Staying Healthy Over 40

By JIM NELSON

American Media, Inc.

NEVER GET SICK

Complete Guide to Staying Healthy Over 40

Copyright © 2005 AMI Books, Inc.

Cover design: Carlos Plaza

Interior design: Debbie Browning

ISBN: 0-9754950-3-8

First printing: February 2005

Printed in the United States of America

10 9 8 7 6 5 4 3 2 1

CHAPTER 1

The Back 40

How did this happen?

One day you were ambling along without a care in the world, turning cartwheels and partying like there was no tomorrow and ...

Suddenly it was tomorrow.

Suddenly that suit didn't fit right anymore, that skirt needed to be let out, the passions of youth gave way to the cares of adulthood.

And before you knew it people were

showering you with black balloons, black crepe, Geritol and a host of other gag gifts as you passed to the dark netherside of 40.

Suddenly you heard the nasty bleep of mortality. Suddenly a scandalously young and ruinously passionate former president was having a heart bypass. Suddenly the knees ached, the belt didn't fit, the hair was falling out and you were no longer a member of a desired demographic. You began to have nightmares about those lime green pants with white belts your grandfather wore back in the 1960s. Or was it one of those frightful leisure suits from the 1970s?

Whatever the image, it didn't seem to fit your own self-perception. As Diane Wiest's character said in the film *Parenthood*:

"I can't be a grandmother — I was at Woodstock, for God's sake!"

Welcome to Life After 40.

Look on the bright side: 20,000 years ago our caveman forefathers (and mothers) were lucky to make it to age 26 before some horrible fate befell them. Unhealed wounds, childbirth, the accumulation of the effects from dozens of incurable diseases, the loss of teeth and a hundred other maladies that today seem banal and easily remedied plagued humans until just recently and kept the population down and life exceedingly short.

Even in 1900, in fact, life expectancy at birth was just 46.3 years for men and 48.0 years for women. As of 2001, life expectancy had risen to 74.4 years for men and 79.8 years for women. The discovery of antibiotics, increased affluence, advances in medicine and nutrition, and other factors have added decades and decades to our lives.

But those advances have led to a paradox: We're living longer lives, but are we living *healthier* lives?

Processed fatty and sugary foods and a decline in exercise as more and more people left the hard work of the farm for the relative ease of urban settings and lifestyles have led to an epidemic of obesity and sharp rises in the incidences of diseases such as diabetes. And whole new areas of medicine have opened up in response to the increase in longevity; because we're living longer, we're seeing more of the cancers and other diseases that have their onset after age 40 or 50 — diseases that death itself forestalled 100 years ago.

Despite the increase in longevity, are we, as a society, healthy? Statistics indicate that the answer is no — that many of us squander what could be healthy extra years on a plethora of bad choices and then look to medicine to salvage our diseased bodies.

We don't exercise enough, we eat poorly, and tobacco and excessive alcohol consumption continue to take their toll.

"Poor eating habits, lack of exercise and smoking are to blame for more than a third of all deaths in the United States" was how one recent news story summed up a report by the U.S. Centers for Disease Control and Prevention.

While the report found tobacco to be the No. 1 killer in the United States, "Poor diet and lack of physical activity, taken together because of their impact on heart disease, stroke and other cardiovascular conditions, was a close second, causing 400,000 deaths" in the year 2000.

The situation calls to mind the famous saying by Cary Grant: "If I had known I was going to live so long, I would have taken better care of myself."

Because most consequences of poor health

choices made during our youth and relative youth — smoking, drinking, overeating, lack of exercise — don't begin to show up until one is past age 40, that age is used for the starting point for this book.

Science and our own empirical evidence tells us that things start to run south at about age 40. Muscle tone sags, it's harder to keep weight off, your sex drive may take a dive — in short, we can't do all the things at 40 or 50 or 60 that we could at half those ages.

But this book has been written to show that we can live healthier, happier, and even longer, lives. No matter your age, no matter your lifestyle history, there are things you can do starting right now — in diet, in exercise, in attitude readjustment — that will begin paying dividends in your overall health right now and, most importantly, 20 and 30 years down the road.

Let *Never Get Sick* be your companion on the rest of your journey through life, a guide to the roads better taken, as well as to the roads better left alone!

CHAPTER 2

Death Don't Have No Mercy

Wouldn't it be great if we had the same body tone at ages 40, 50, 60 and beyond that we have at 21?

No battle of the bulge, no aching knees, no stiff backs, no arrhythmias or reading glasses, no senility, no need for Viagra or calcium or other supplements aimed at restoring that which once — was it really so long ago? — coursed naturally through our youthful veins.

Wouldn't it be great to remain, as Dylan Thomas put it in his masterful poem Fern Hill: *"green and carefree, famous among the barns/About the happy yard and singing as the farm was home/In the sun that is young once only ... "*

But, no.

We are mortal. Finite. We grow old. We lament, like Thomas:

"Oh as I was young and easy in the mercy of his means,

Time held me green and dying

Though I sang in my chains like the sea."

But it's not just time that does this dirty work.

Aging involves a million tiny little processes insidiously at work in our bodies. Miniscule little misses among the billions of chemical reactions and syntheses going on all day and all night account, most experts agree, for what ultimately manifests themselves in aching joints, wrinkles, thickening lenses and all the other hallmarks of age.

What is aging? "A process of gradual and spontaneous change, resulting in maturation through childhood, puberty and young adulthood and then decline through middle and late age," says the definition in the *Merck Manual of Geriatrics*.

Within that process, that "gradual and spontaneous change," aging is at work. Two main theories vie in trying to pin down exactly why this process of change can make our bodies go from hale and hearty to fizzled and bent over the course of 60 or 70 years.

The Error Catastrophe Theory, also known as the Orgel Catastrophe Theory, holds that aging is the result of a lifetime of errors which accumulate each time cells divide.

The theory posits that our DNA and RNA, the basic building blocks of life, lose just a little something each time cells replicate and over time the exactly coded sequences gather enough miniscule mistakes to make a difference. Each new cell runs a little off-kilter, until over time these accumulated mistakes cause breakdowns in the operation of the body and mind. Performance of individual cells and then cell groups — tissues — becomes fuzzy, impaired; mutations increase.

"Maintenance of the structural integrity

of DNA is critical not only for cell survival but also for the transfer of correct genetic information to daughter cells," says one description of the theory. "Alterations in the fidelity of DNA polymerase alpha could result in a progressive degradation in information transfer during DNA synthesis, which would eventually affect a wide range of cellular components during aging ...

"Mutations, which are harmless in a first time, may become deleterious when their effect is combined with other insignificant changes in the internal organization of a living entity, just because, for instance, there is a threshold in the number of these mutations and changes, from which a metabolic function is impaired."

In other words, a bunch of tiny and almost imperceptible errors in the transfer of our genetic code from mother cell to baby cells adds up over time to create large trouble, as the coding becomes hard to read. In time, says the theory, the operation of a group of cells, then a group of tissues, then an organ won't function well because of this accumulation of errors.

"Although data suggest that older organisms have altered proteins reflective of such genetic changes," says the *Merck Manual*, "this theory does little to explain most observed age-related changes."

Another theory has gained more and more credibility over the years, as elements of it seem to be proved in lab and other experiments.

Known as the Loose Cannon Theory, it posits that through a body process known as oxidation — a continuous and important job throughout the body associated with breathing and moving and just living — highly reactive molecules called free radicals break off.

Single atoms, these free radicals have an unpaired electron attached to them. Needing a mate, these molecules bounce through the body grabbing an electron wherever it can be found — from cell walls, for instance, or even DNA strands.

As one writer put it, "Simply eating and breathing can cause free radicals." And over time, this stealing of electrons causes damage within cells.

As with Orgel's catastrophic theory, the functions of cells and then groups of cells begin to wither and break down. "Tissues degrade" is how one writer put it. "Disease sets in. An excess of free radicals has been cited in the development of cardiovascular disease, Alzheimer's disease, Parkinson's disease and cancer. Aging itself has been defined as a gradual accumulation of free radical damage."

And scientists have taken note of the effect of free radicals. "Considerable evidence suggests that oxidative damage increases with age," notes the *Merck Manual*.

Besides those tiny but inexorable and bizarre activities going on inside our bodies every minute of every day, our bodies also tend to break down out of simple disuse.

As children, the simple acts of running and jumping and playing hour after hour builds our muscles and bones. As we head into middle age, we generally are less active — we become bound to desks, car seats and sofas as work and the pressures of everyday living — the kids, the mortgage, the job — leave little room or even inclination to jump around like a bunch of whacked-out kangaroos.

"People lose 20 percent to 40 percent of their muscle — and, along with it, their strength — as they age," concludes one report from the National Institute on Aging. "Scientists have found that a major reason people lose muscle is because they stop doing everyday activities that use muscle power, not just because they grow older. Lack of use lets muscles waste away."

Lack of use also compounds another major factor in aging — the throttling down of our metabolisms, the mechanism by which we burn calories.

Experts say we lose 5 percent of metabolic function every decade past 40, so that a resting metabolic rate — the rate your body burns calories while at rest — of 1,200 calories a day at age 40 can decline to a resting rate of just 1,140 at age 50.

That means either the calories stay — or you have to pump up your activities to burn those extra 60 calories a day. But, as noted before, life tends to intervene, leading to a pack-on of extra flab as those daily 60 calories accrue and multiply.

"As we age, our lives become more complicated, whether it's with children, with work or with aging parents, so we have less time really to be more physically active and pay attention to what we're eating," notes Dr. Madelyn Fernstrom, director of the University of Pittsburgh Medical Center Weight Management Center.

"Food is available 24 hours a day, seven days a week, in large portions that are relatively economical. So food is always around and we tend to have more mindless eating and cut down on activities."

Genetics, thyroid function and muscle mass affect your rate of metabolism, says Dr. Pamela Peeke, an assistant professor of medicine at the University of Maryland School of Medicine. While there's not much one can do about one's genetics — not now, anyway — Peeke notes again that lifestyle issues have a lot to do with a slowing metabolism.

"Muscle is very metabolically active and you don't want to lose it," she said. "What's happening is if you don't use it, you lose it and in your 40s you don't just lose it, it melts.

"A typical man can lose over the course of age 30 through age 50 anywhere between five and 10 pounds of muscle mass. A woman could definitely lose that — that's a

given because she, through repeated diet-
ing and decreased physical activity, will
lose that."

Of course, loss of muscle begins with
some of the normal wear-and-tear of living.
That ill-advised slide you took into third
base at the company picnic; those many
tweaks and twinges you felt when lifting
your toddler; that spill from a bike when
you were showing Ma how good you were
with no hands, even that three-week bender
in college when you were 20 — hey, life happens — and beyond all that intra-cell high
science regarding electrons and protons
and God knows what, the effects of
mishaps, tiny and large, accrue over time in
our muscles, bones and cartilage.

Not to mention all of those triple-bacon-
cheeseburger cholesterol bombs and those
hundreds of thousands of blessedly empty
calories you've trusted your body with over
the years, the effects of which are coming
home to roost in your thighs, buttocks and
other highly visible places.

Why mention all of this?

Because while time holds us "green and
dying," by understanding the processes

affecting our bodies we can find ways to sing in our chains not just like the sea, but like the Mormon Tabernacle Choir.

Or maybe like Robert Plant, even.

We also mention these theories on aging because much of today's treatment of the causes and symptoms of aging revolves around the effort to rid the body of free radicals by the use of natural or supplemental antioxidants — substances that swallow and neutralize these free radicals. And besides that, there are other supplements, exercises, lifestyle choices and diet factors that can help restore vigor. Part of *Never Get Sick* is about understanding what can, and what cannot, be done to maintain our bodies or even to reclaim some of our youthful plasticity.

Outside of genetic factors, most experts point to lifestyle choices as the main culprit in unhealthy aging, a fact underlined by the staid and no-frills *Merck Manual*. "Most age-related biological functions peak at (less than) 30 years of age and may gradually decline in a linear fashion," the manual states. "Although this later decline may be critical during stress, it has no effect on daily activity. Thus, disease, rather than normal aging, is the prime determinant of functional loss in old age. Many decrements reportedly caused by aging are more often attributable to lifestyle, behavior, diet or environment, which can be modified ...

"The effects of aging may be less dramatic than previously thought and healthier, more vigorous aging may be possible for many persons."

Ultimately, the only cure for life remains death, but there are ways in which you can age right, age vigorously, to borrow Merck's phrase, and at the very least freeze the clock and get yourself on the right track to good health — or simply maintain the good shape you're already in.

CHAPTER 3

Shake It ...

So, how to age vigorously?

One key is to exercise, exercise and then exercise some more.

Whew.

It's true. Though study after study bemoans our indolence and overall tendency to be couch potatoes, health experts agree that one key and undeniable factor in extending one's life is exercise — which can override other factors, including genetic makeup.

"Exercise ... tends to lower blood pressure, decreasing the risk of heart attack and stroke, and trims the chance of becoming obese or developing non-insulin-dependent diabetes mellitus," says one report.

"Regular physical activity has also been linked with lower rates of certain kinds of cancer. In general, exercise extends longevity by diminishing the risk of a variety of different ailments."

"Studies repeatedly show that regular, moderate-to-vigorous exercise can help prevent or delay the onset of hypertension, obesity, heart disease, osteoporosis and the falls that lead to hip fracture," another study noted.

Research on twins "is proving that regular exercise can help extend the life span of every individual, regardless of their individual genetic makeup," one study reported in the *Journal of the American Medical Association* concluded. "Leisure-time physical activity is associated with reduced mortality, even after genetic and other familial factors are taken into account."

The study on twins designated "those who reported exercising for at least 30 minutes at least six times per month" as "conditioning exercisers, while those reporting less regular exercise were labeled occasional exercisers. Individuals reporting no regular exercise were considered sedentary by the researchers.

"The investigators found that individual twins who engaged in vigorous conditioning exercise were able to reduce their risk of death by an average of 43 percent compared with sedentary types. And they found that even occasional exercisers were able to reduce their mortality risk by 29 percent compared with non-exercisers.

"Even though twins share highly similar genetic and familial backgrounds ... those who exercised managed to reap the health benefits of their ongoing activity, while those avoiding activity suffered relative declines. The researchers say their findings suggest that regular exercise is a preventative factor for premature mortality, independent of genetic influences."

And even if your idea of exercise is walking across the street to get the mail or bringing in the groceries, and you're already past age 40, research suggests overwhelmingly that it's never too late to begin a regular program.

It doesn't matter when you start — or if you already have a chronic condition related to inactivity.

"A lifetime of regular aerobic and resistance exercise is 'the ideal,' " one study said. "However, the initiation of exercise in adulthood is also beneficial ... although vigorous exercise may provide more cardiovascular benefits, moderate physical activity is nearly as beneficial and conveys less risk of injury. In other words, any form of exercise — even in advanced age — can serve as primary prevention to maintain good physical health."

One recent study of older men found that a regular exercise program, begun after decades of inactivity, completely restored the loss of cardiovascular capacity that inactivity had bestowed upon them.

"Everyone said they felt as good as they had ever felt in their lives," said the study's architect, Dr. Darren McGuire of the University of Texas Southwestern Medical Center. "This study shows it's never too late to get physically fit, even if you've been sedentary for years."

However, Dr. McGuire — and other experts at the National Institute on Aging and elsewhere — cautions that persons who have not been working out need to start with an easy program and slowly increase the amount and intensity of exercise over a period of months.

"Your first target should be 30 minutes three times a week," Dr. McGuire says. "Your ultimate target is 30 minutes five to seven times a week, but any exercise is better than no exercise. It's never too late to get physically fit — even if you've been sedentary for years."

Another analysis of 37 different studies showed that exercise may actually slow the effects of aging on cardiovascular systems. The studies, which overall involved 720 adults ages 46 to 90, showed that people who exercised at least three times a week for 30 minutes at a time and achieved at least 80 percent of their maximum oxygen consumption were able to slow the cardiovascular decline that comes with aging.

Lifelong exercisers did not show more benefits from their workouts than those who had been working out for a shorter time — "suggesting that improvements can be made in less than four months and then maintained after that point," the analysis said. The outcome was the same for walkers, joggers and bicyclists.

Another study of people in their 70s found that regular exercisers regained an average of 22 percent of the lung capacity that had been lost due to inactivity. "This achievement effectively restored the exercisers' daily lung function to levels experienced in their 50s," the study found.

Such success was also found in the area of muscle recovery.

One study done in 1994 found that people who were age 75 and older recovered 21 percent of their muscle strength after three months of resistance training. The authors of the study believe the recovery was due to expansion of existing muscle fiber.

"When you have enough muscle, it can mean the difference between being able to get up from a chair by yourself and having to wait for someone to help you get up," says the report from the NIA. "That's true for younger adults as well as for people ages 90 and older. Very small changes in muscle size, changes that you can't even see, can make a big difference in your being able to live and do things on your own."

Another report had similar findings. While noting that there is some loss of muscle and cardiovascular ability with age no matter if a person exercises or not, "The loss in muscle mass and the decreases in strength and endurance associated with inactivity are totally reversible with subsequent conditioning."

The report, titled *Prescription For Longevity*, noted that we lose 30 percent to 40 percent of our muscle mass between ages 30 and 70 — and suggested a "minimum" expenditure of 1,000 calories per week "above baseline sedentary levels" for most adults, the equivalent of walking four miles a day, five times a week.

While that may sound like a lot, the report actually preferred that Americans exercise more — the equivalent of jogging that 20 miles a week!

And speaking of jogging — yeah, we know, it sucks — a Danish study found that joggers "are significantly less likely than non-runners to die of any cause."

A study of 4,600 men ages 20 to 79 found that regular joggers were 63 percent less likely than other men to die over the course of five years. However, occasional joggers did not have a lower death risk than non-joggers.

"Researchers note that while jogging has become increasingly popular over the past 30 years, there is some public concern over reports of people dying while jogging," the study said. "However, despite public misconceptions, this study shows that regular joggers boast a significantly lower risk of dying. The joggers' lower death rate could be a direct effect of the exercise or the men may have led more healthy lifestyles in general."

So if you want to stay healthy after 40, exercise is a must. If you have little history of exercising and staying fit, the task of simply beginning can seem daunting — especially to someone who's already over 50. But, as is noted above, there are many ways to exercise.

Walk up the stairs instead of taking the elevator, ride a bike, walk, play a little tennis — it's the engagement of muscle and the cardiovascular that matters. And it's simple to make exercising an everyday part of your life.

"Go for brisk walks," advises the NIA. "Ride a bike. Dance. And don't stop doing physical tasks around the house and in the yard. Trim the hedges without a power tool. Climb stairs. Rake leaves.

"You can combine activities — for example, walking uphill and raking leaves build both endurance and some of your muscles at the same time. Or you can start an exercise program that makes sure you do the right types of activities."

As for getting started on a workout program, "You should stop thinking in terms of 'exercise' and think in terms of movements," advises Dr. Bess Marcus, director of the Physical Activity Research Center at the Brown University School of Medicine.

"For instance, if you're gardening, that counts. If you walk briskly around the mall while you're shopping rather than lollygagging, that counts.

"You can also fit an activity into a spot that's already taken up by a daily activity. So if you watch the news every night at 6 p.m., watch it while riding a stationary bike or walking on the treadmill. If you read the paper every morning, read it while working out on your home machine. If you'd rather spend your free time curled up with a book, get a book on tape and take it with you on a walk around the neighborhood.

"We need to make sure that getting our activity in is high enough up in our thinking that it's one of the things we multitask with."

Take baby steps. "The first step is to get at least 30 minutes of activity that makes you breathe harder, on most or all days of the week," the NIA says.

"That's called 'endurance activity' because it builds your stamina. That way you can keep doing the things you need to do and the things you like to do. If you can't be active for 30 minutes all at once, get at least 10 minutes of endurance activity at a time. If you choose to do 10-minute sessions, make sure that they add up to a total of 30 minutes at the end of the day.

"Even a moderate level of sustained activity helps. One doctor described the right level of effort this way: 'If you can talk without any trouble at all, your activity is probably too easy. If you can't talk at all, it's too hard.'"

Exercise helps stave off a particular muscle-wasting disease that afflicts the elderly, as well.

The disease, called sarcopenia, results in the loss of muscle mass. "Older people with significant sarcopenia can have difficulty caring for themselves and frequently need to enter a nursing home for constant monitoring," notes a report from the International Longevity Center-USA.

A study done over two years by New Mexico authorities found that 13 percent of men and 8 percent of women under the age of 70 suffered from sarcopenia — with the percentages of the afflicted rising to 17.5 percent at age 75. But strength training has been found to reduce frailty and stave off the disease.

"Men and women who trained for eight to 12 weeks showed average increases in muscle strength ranging from 113 percent to 174 percent," the report noted. The training was not especially rigorous — just a few sets of lifting each week brought good results.

Exercise brings other benefits. In a University of Wisconsin study, 60 women were interviewed in an effort to find out if a person's level of activity could be linked to their state of mind.

The study compared responses from more sedentary women with their peers who still went out of their way to walk, climb stairs, shop or clean house. "The women with hustle felt happier, healthier, more socially connected and more pleased with their environments than their sedentary peers — even when their health and living conditions were otherwise nearly identical," the study found.

The study's author concluded: "In the long term, older adults hurt their health more by not exercising than by exercising."

And a study examining the exercise habits among older people who suffered from chronic lung problems found that routine workouts helped stave off the physical decline that comes with age — and also put at bay declines in memory and other brain functions.

The participants in the study, average age 65, did aerobics for 10 weeks. They exercised for an hour daily for five weeks, then cut back to three hour-long aerobic sessions weekly.

Comparing the battery of emotional, cognitive and physical tests given before and after the 10-week workout regimen, researchers reported that the overall scores improved. Another round of tests, done a year later, found that those who had continued to exercise also maintained their physical and cognitive abilities — while those who stopped exercising slid back and declined in their scores.

"We found that the people who continued to exercise remained stable and it was the people who stopped exercising or exercised irregularly who showed a decline," said the study's lead author, Charles Emery, a psychology professor at Ohio State University.

Besides all of the other life-giving and sustaining benefits of exercise, regular seat-producing workouts can make you exude youth. Exercise builds another muscle — the heart — which pumps more vigorously. Blood vessels are less likely to be dumping sites for harmful plaque, and from the aorta to the capillaries that wend through our skin, blood is bringing oxygen and nutrients to every organ and every cell in our bodies. "Emerging research suggests that most of your susceptibility to wrinkles, flab, muscle loss and chronic health problems such as heart disease and osteoporosis can be managed through exercise, diet and even what you slather on your face," notes one writer.

Some experts say that age 35 is, at the very least, the time to start working to retain bone density and muscle mass through exercise. "For every decade of inactivity after your 30s, you'll lose 10 percent of your muscle mass," says one report in *Prevention* magazine. "You'll also gain fat and weight even if you don't change your eating habits, because calorie-hungry muscle burns more calories per pound than any other kind of tissue." In other words, using your muscles can expedite weight loss.

How can you stave off the loss of muscle mass? Pump some iron. It not only builds muscle, it's also good for strengthening bones. One study of 25 women found that those who started strength training before they were in their 40s had bigger gains in bone density — especially important in women — than those who didn't start until their 50s or later. Some experts advise twice-weekly workouts of weight or resistance training to build muscles.

And you don't have to be like Arnold Schwarzenegger to pump iron. Just start out with small weights — a couple of one-pounders will do — and do sets of 10 to 15 lifts and curls twice a week. You can even use anything lying around the house — a heavy book will do the trick. After several weeks, move up to three pounds and do the same repetitions. Try to increase the weight you're pumping every few weeks.

Resistance training is easy and requires no special equipment, either. You can do sets of push-ups — remember to start slow and easy if you haven't worked out for awhile — or simply lean and push against a wall for 10 seconds at a time.

Aerobics is another great way to get into shape and stay there. Find an aerobics class in your area, or simply begin by jumping rope, bicycling or walking. "In your 30s take advantage of the fact that your joints can still handle high-intensity aerobic exercises, such as jumping rope and jogging," says one writer. For people in their 30s, "Whatever aerobic regimen you choose, aim for 30 to 60 minutes at a sweat-breaking pace four or five times a week."

By age 45, "you may have lost enough muscle to have slowed your metabolism, which means weight gain and heart troubles are real risks," one writer notes. It may be time to sign up for "integrated training," which combines aerobics with muscle- and bone-building strength training. If you're too pressed for time between family and career obligations, try to combine family time and training time by riding a bicycle, walking or jogging together — or even by renting an exercise video and working out at home with the kids.

Male or female, it's never too late to start building muscle and bone density and increasing muscle tone and the flow of blood to the skin. However, experts caution that if you are now age 55 or older and haven't exercised strenuously for some time, it's best to have a checkup with your doctor before you begin any kind of vigorous workout program. Hidden health problems such as heart disease, a heart condition or diabetes need to be ruled out before beginning a strenuous exercise program.

But people ages 55 and older are the people who most benefit from exercise. One study of 173 inactive, overweight women ages 50 to 75 discovered that the women who began an exercise program of 45 minutes, five days a week lost 4 percent of their total body fat. And that hard-to-eliminate belly fat, which older women are especially prone to develop, was also reduced — as was the risk of developing osteoporosis.

So get up and shake it a little. Move that thing. You've got nothing to lose — except some weight.

CHAPTER 4

... But Don't Break It

OK, OK, I'll exercise.

But how much is enough?

Well, it's becoming apparent that the intensity of your workout is linked to the benefits of the workout.

It's not a matter of no pain, no gain, because, as noted previously, simple aerobic activities and weight training have obvious health benefits. But studies are showing that weight loss, muscle building and other benefits of exercise can be amped even further by more rigorous workouts.

But you don't have to start competing in triathlons.

Dr. Pamela Peeke of the University of Maryland says that all that's required to cut those extra calories gained because of a slowing metabolism as we age — which over time can add 20, 30, 40 or more pounds — is a little more exertion.

"The kind of physical activity that people are choosing to do in their 40s is nowhere near as intense as it's supposed to be," she told WebMD. "So to get over that metabolic speed bump we ask for an increase in intensity on the part of these happy campers.

"What does that mean? Instead of walking on the flat, throw in some hills. Ramp up the resistance in your resistance training or, for that matter, the resistance on a cross-trainer. It's all the same."

"Even if we do have a small, let's say, biological sabotage built in, it does not mean everyone is destined to gain weight as they grow older," adds the University of Pittsburgh's Madelyn Fernstrom.

"It's sort of an old wives' tale that you'll gain 30 or 40 pounds as you continue through middle age — it can easily happen, but it's very easy to offset the change in metabolic rate.

"For most people that's going to be 100 calories a day approximately. If you are over-consuming just that 100 calories, you can gain 10 pounds a year if you are out of sync 100 calories a day."

"People at 50 find themselves getting into a more sedentary lifestyle," said Dr. Alfred Morris, an exercise scientist and assistant director for health and fitness at the National Defense University. "Their metabolism slows down. They lose lean body mass and gain fat."

But, "with regular workouts, they can maintain their cardiovascular efficiency and protect the lean body mass they already have."

A little more oomph — a mad dash at the end of a jog, a few more repetitions with the weights and an extra quarter-mile on the walk — can add to the intensity of the workout and burn those extra calories that can sink us, as well as further sharpen our heart rates and other biological functions.

The *Prescription For Longevity* report mentioned previously, which urged us all to do the equivalent of jogging 20 miles a week, is in agreement on the greater health benefits in heavier, rather than just any, level of exercise.

"These findings support the current view of the medical community that, although light exercise seems to have some value, moderate to vigorous activity such as jogging is now considered more favorable for health."

And studies back up this view. One, an examination of 9,376 male civil servants in Britain who were ages 45 to 64, found that the subjects had to engage in exercise classified as vigorous — swimming, football, hockey, etc. — twice a week in order to enjoy a lower rate of heart attack.

Heart-attack rates were found to be reduced by 67 percent in these men and the mortality rate for the vigorous exercisers was reduced by 80 to 90 percent compared to the men who worked out less or not at all.

There are studies for and about women, as well.

One, Women Walking For Health and Fitness, split 59 previously sedentary women ages 20 to 40 on four different exercise paths. Sixteen of the women walked 4.8 kilometers a day, five days a week, at a speed of 8 kilometers per hour. Twelve other women walked the same distance and as often, but at a 6.4 kilometer-per-hour pace. Eighteen of the women moseyed along at 4.8 kilometers per hour and the final 13 women served as controls for the study.

After six months, the fastest walkers showed the greatest improvements in their cardiovascular health — and all three groups had comparable drops in body fat and improvement in levels of the "good" cholesterol — HDLs.

Though any exercise is better for your health than none, the jury is divided as to how much added benefit — if any — results from more intense physical activity.

Some studies support the idea that pushing the envelope is better for you than just plodding along just enough to get your heart rate up.

One study, performed at Ohio University, featured a group of men ages 60 to 75 who were split into two groups of nine — one group performed resistance training over the course of 16 weeks and the other was used as a control.

Not surprisingly, lung capacity and muscle strength improved "significantly" for those who did the resistance training. "Training programs for older individuals should not differ considerably from those prescribed for young people," commented one expert about the report. "The same relative resistance needed to make a young person's muscle respond is the same needed for a person decades older. Any person, young or old, looking to lose some fat and build some muscle should not procrastinate another day."

In another study, 2,000 men ages 45 to 59 were followed for 10 years. "Initially, none of the men had any evidence of heart disease," said one account of the study. "Exercise was performed and measured by three levels of intensity: low, moderate and high. Low-intensity included walking and bowling. Golf and dancing qualified as moderate-intensity. Running and swimming were in the high-intensity category"

Researchers found that low- and moderate-intensity exercisers were more prone to die prematurely. "Only the highest levels of exercise intensity lowered death rates," said an account of the study.

The results, claims one high-intensity workout advocate, were enough to "destroy" the claim that walking 30 minutes a day was enough to delay heart disease and premature death.

"Long, slow forms of cardio — like walking — is a great place to begin if someone is inactive," the expert wrote. But anaerobic exercise — sprinting, cross-country skiing, etc. — "is the most productive form of exercise and it should be a part of every fitness routine. However, anaerobic exercise is the most dangerous form of exercise and physician clearance is a must. A progressive buildup program — from low, to moderate, to high-intensity — is necessary to prevent injury."

Dr. Alfred Morris says older athletes should be aware of their bodies' changes and work slower. As the body ages, muscles and tendons can lose their stretching ability and become more likely to strain and tear.

"One way is just to start the activity slowly," Dr. Morris advises. "As your body starts to feel good with it, gear up to higher intensities."

If you do feel pain while working out, stop. If you need to, switch to another activity — do a week of swimming instead of running, for instance.

And keep in mind that, as mentioned above, the jury is still out regarding the ultimate benefits of intense versus low or moderate workouts.

One study says the ultimate level of exercise needed to prevent heart disease differs according to age and fitness levels.

"Brisk walking, at 3 to 4 miles per hour, would not require much effort for a young, physically fit man, relative to his fitness because he is highly fit," said Harvard professor I-Min Lee, a lead researcher on the study, which was published in the American Heart Association journal *Circulation.*

"He might perceive this as 'light' exercise.

However, for an older, unfit woman, the same level of activity might require all of her energy. She might perceive this as 'very vigorous' exercise.

Dr. Lee found that even if your current activity doesn't meet current recommendations on exercise levels, you can lower your risk of heart disease by simply exercising as hard as you can — whether that's sprinting laps around the track or walking around the lake.

"The findings can be helpful for older persons who may be unable or unwilling to follow current recommendations," Dr. Lee said. "Don't worry about whether your exertion level corresponds to current recommendations. If you persist at your own rate and become more physically fit, you should then ratchet up your intensity to continue to receive health benefits."

But experts also warn that precautions should be taken to guard against the risk of injury and, down the road, problems such as arthritis.

If you're considering ramping up your current workout or going back to that after-work basketball game you used to enjoy, consider this advice from the American Academy of Orthopedic Surgeons:

- Before starting a sports activity, do sustained muscle stretching and three to five minutes of warmups with a quick jog or on a bike or stationary bicycle.
- Use good equipment, especially good shoes.
- Don't be a "weekend warrior" who plays hard just once or twice a week. Do a half hour of exercise per day on other days of the week. This will help you stay in shape for the more intense workouts, helping prevent injury.
- If you're increasing your workout level, do it in small increments. The 10 percent rule — going from 1 mile, say, to 1.1 miles, instead of suddenly pushing your body to do 3 miles — is a suggested guide.
- Vary your exercise routine with activities that include strength training as well as aerobics.
- Keep you weight at a "reasonable" level to keep stress off your knees.
- Don't overdo it — when it feels like it's time to stop a particular activity due to fatigue, it probably is. Listen to your body.

CHAPTER 5

Never Eat at a Place Called Ma's

It used to be so easy.

Mom made meat and potatoes; you found ways not to eat your carrots and peas, and that food pyramid hanging on the wall of your classroom in sixth grade was heavy on meat and dairy. Cheese, eggs, big juicy steaks, bacon — life was good.

But life was also shorter.

In some ways, we've come a long way in our understanding of nutrition.

As *Health* magazine noted recently, "Scientists used to sneer at the notion that what you eat could influence how you age. But the discovery of little things called antioxidants decades ago changed all that."

Remember free radicals, those bands of dirty, venal brigands within our cells that bop around and force us to age against our will? It's pretty much accepted to various degrees that minerals and vitamins can help rid our cells of these free radicals and limit the damage they do — stopping, or at least slowing down, in effect, the aging process.

But despite all of the discoveries about foods and their properties, we're still hopelessly mired in conflicting information, and arguments for this diet or against that one.

What with Atkins, Pritikin, Hollywood, South Beach, low-carb, high-carb, vegan, vegetarian and a thousand other diets screaming for your attention from magazine and television ads, it's hard to know just what's right — and wrong — when it comes to breakfast, lunch and dinner.

Far from espousing any one plan or "miracle" diet, we're going to keep it simple and tout the Amazing Common Sense Diet (hold the exclamation point, please).

We'll also take a look at several different theories on how to eat, by which we don't mean how to hold chopsticks but how to — so some say — minimize calories by getting away from the three-squares-a-day menu.

But first things first.

Apart from the fads — including the controversial low-carbohydrate diets currently sweeping the nation and changing the very food industry we've come to know and love — experts recommend a sensible, balanced diet based on the reworked "food pyramid" of carbohydrates, proteins and fats. In addition, some experts recommend supplemental vitamins and minerals.

But junk food — potato and other chips, sodas, cookies, fatty fried foods — are on almost every diet expert's list of things not to do when trying to eat healthy.

We are what we eat — or don't eat. And when it comes to staying healthy and adding years to our lives, no other factor — except smoking — may determine our ability to stay healthy.

According to a report from the American Institute for Cancer Research (AICR), "many cancer cases" can be prevented worldwide each year simply by altering lifestyles.

"Experts found that 30 to 40 percent of all cases of cancers could be prevented if people would make recommended dietary choices, keep physically active and maintain a healthy body weight."

The AICR recommended the following guidelines for cancer prevention:

- **Choose a diet rich in a variety of plant-based foods**
- **Eat plenty of vegetables and fruits**
- **Maintain a healthy weight and be physically active**
- **Drink alcohol only in moderation, if at all (more on this later)**
- **Select foods low in fat and salt**
- **Prepare and store food safely**

In espousing the above guidelines, the AICR noted the shift in thinking from the fats-starch-and-protein gut bombs Mom used to make to the new thinking governing nutrition today.

"Many of us grew up as 'meat and potatoes' people," the report notes. "As a result, eating more plant-based foods is probably a new idea. In our lifetimes, a wealth of information has come to light about the ways in which foods can affect our health. We know that by choosing to eat more foods that come from plants and fewer that come from animals, we can benefit our health in many ways, including helping to prevent cancer and heart disease, maintain a healthy weight and promote digestion.

"We know that plant substances found in vegetables and fruits can help prevent the cell damage that, over time, can lead to the weakening of body tissues such as skin, organs and vessels, and disease such as cancer.

"Getting enough calcium and vitamin D can help prevent osteoporosis, the leading cause of bone fractures in older adults. The B vitamins folate, B6 and B12 may help reduce the risk of heart disease and stroke. Early studies show these vitamins could possibly delay a decline in brain activities like concentration, reason and memory that may come with age."

After analyzing the alternatives, the

International Longevity Center-USA issued a report that also recommends a diet rich in fruits and vegetables. Calories from fat, the center said, should be no more than 30 percent of total caloric intake.

"Dietary deficiencies are a well-known risk factor for many diseases, including age-related diseases such as cancer, cardiovascular disease and osteoporosis," the center said in its report. "Epidemiological data on dietary intakes indicate that in persons whose diet is rich in fruits and vegetables, the risk of a variety of cancers is lowered by one-half."

The National Institute on Aging has detailed its recommended dietary guidelines as well in its own attempt to show people how to live healthy lives.

"Choose many different healthy foods," the NIA says. "Pick those that are lower in fat, especially saturated fat (mostly in foods that come from animals), and cholesterol. Eat and drink only small amounts of sugary or salty foods and alcoholic drinks, if you drink them at all. Avoid 'empty' calories as much as you can. These are foods like sodas, potato chips and cookies that have a lot of calories, but not many nutrients."

Scientists are also recognizing the importance of fiber in a healthy diet. Eating enough fiber, the undigested portion of grain, fruits and vegetables, is key to maintaining a healthy digestive track, helping waste products move through more efficiently and preventing such conditions as constipation and painful diverticulitis. Some experts recommend that a person eat 20 to 35 grams of fiber daily and also recommend that it come from the food you eat, not supplements. To achieve the recommended amount of fiber you should:

- **Eat cooked dry beans and lentils regularly**
- **Eat fruits and vegetables with the skin on if possible**
- **Eat whole fruit instead of drinking the juice – the fiber is in the fruit**
- **Eat whole-grain breads and cereals**
- **Drink plenty of fluids to keep everything moving smoothly through your system**

So you really were supposed to eat your vegetables. Who knew?

And not only that, you were supposed to be eating a lot more of them than even Mom was pushing.

How does all this translate into a regular

diet that can keep us healthy whether we're 30, 40, 50 or beyond?

Choosing a diet rich in plant-based foods — this means grains, vegetables, roots such as potatoes, and fruits — doesn't mean you have to be a vegetarian. It does mean that the old equation of — let's be honest here — 80 percent meat, 15 percent potatoes and 5 percent vegetables you couldn't sneak to your dog is out the window.

Here's one recommendation. The U.S. Department of Agriculture's food guide pyramid contains five major food groups people should eat every day. Using that pyramid, the NIA recommends the following servings and amounts per day:

Grains. *6 to 11 servings.* In the course of a day, this could be a slice of bread, half a bagel, a half-cup of rice or pasta, a half-cup of cooked cereal and a cup of ready-to-eat cereal.

Vegetables. *3 to 5 servings a day.* One serving is equal to half a cup of chopped vegetables or a cup of leafy raw vegetables.

Fruits. *2 to 4 servings.* One serving is one medium melon wedge, one piece of fruit or three-fourths of a cup of juice. One-quarter cup of dried fruit also counts as a serving.

Milk, yogurt and cheese. *2 to 3 servings.* A serving is equal to one cup of yogurt or milk or one-and-a-half to two ounces of cheese or two cups of cottage cheese.

Meat, poultry, fish, dry beans, eggs and nuts. *2 to 3 servings (totaling 5 to 7 ounces per day).* One serving is two to three ounces of cooked lean meat or one-half cup of tuna fish or one-half cup of cooked beans or tofu, one egg, one-third of a cup of nuts or two tablespoons of peanut butter.

Combining the wisdom of "the leading gerontologists and nutrition scientists," *Health* magazine put together "the ultimate anti-aging meal." It looks like this:

First course: *Roaster butternut squash soup with toasted almonds and pomegranate molasses*

Main course: *Grilled marinated blue fin tuna steaks with asparagus, oregano and tomato confit; roasted-garlic mashed potatoes* (hey — meat and potatoes!)

Salad: *Spinach, mushrooms, beets, goat cheese and pecans*

Dessert: *Three scoops of sorbet served with cranberry-and-pistachio biscotti*

After-dinner drink: *Green tea*

Cheryl Forberg, author of *Stop the Clock! Cooking,* says the ideal anti-aging meal — and we're equating not aging with attaining great overall health — would be "a piece of wild salmon, a large bowl of dark-green leafy vegetables and steamed broccoli."

Catherine Downey, associate dean of the National College for Naturopathic Medicine, likes what she calls a "3-2-1" formula.

"Eat three servings of vegetables, two pieces of fruit and a whole grain — for example, a cup of brown rice or oatmeal — every day," Downey says, adding that one cup equals one serving.

The point is to maximize the amount of vitamins, minerals and fiber you can get from your food without having to resort to supplements (more on supplements later) while also limiting the fats that have been implicated in the origins of heart disease and some cancers.

And of course, there's more to eating than eating. There's drinking, too.

For a long time, experts have recommended drinking eight 8-ounce glasses of water — or its equivalent — per day. The equivalent can be found in juice, milk, even soup. We lose water every moment of the day and replacing the water in our bodies is essential for balancing salts and minerals and maintaining proper cell function.

The National Institute on Aging recommends in a report that older people drink water or its equivalent whether they're thirsty or not. "Don't wait until you feel thirsty to start drinking," its report says. "With age you may lose some of your sense of thirst. In addition, medicine can sometimes cause you to lose fluids. If you are drinking enough, your urine will be pale yellow. If it is a bright or dark yellow, you need to drink more liquids."

On the other hand, intake of salt needs to be limited to 2,400 milligrams per day — about one teaspoon. Though the perils of too much salt have been well-described in recent decades — excessive sodium is implicated in high blood pressure and other ailments — the fact remains that your body needs sodium for healthy blood, muscles and nerves. However, people overall eat too much salt, especially from processed foods such as chips and canned soups.

Fat, as well, has been fingered as the cause

of many of our nutritional ills in recent decades. That still hasn't prevented the developed world — and the United States in particular — from overindulging in fatty processed and fast foods, but the fact is that we do need some fats. Fats provide the oils that protect our skin and hair, and also contain some essential vitamins. Fat provides energy as well. But too much fat, especially saturated fats, can lead to deposits in the blood vessels and lead to heart disease.

As mentioned previously, the NIA recommends that no more than 30 percent of calories come from fat — 53 grams in the typical 1,600-calorie-per-day diet an adult woman might eat (a teaspoon of butter or margarine, for instance, has about 4 grams of fat).

Besides staying away from those triple bacon-cheeseburgers at the drive-thru and keeping your mitts out of those big bags of nacho cheese chips, there are ways to cut down on fat intake:

- Choose lean, skinless cuts of meat, fish and poultry
- Use unsaturated oils for cooking
- Avoid frying foods — broil, roast, bake, microwave or stir-fry instead

● **Season foods with lemon, herbs or spices instead of butter**

But wait ... there's more.

Besides the many diets vying for our attention (read: money), a whole genre of ideas telling us how to eat has reared its head as well.

Some experts are certain that when you eat and how much you eat are almost as important as what you eat.

To fast or not to fast? To eat small meals all day or to stick with our three-squares-a-day routine, just like Ma wanted us to?

There's no real answer here. Just, uh, food for thought.

Let's start with fasting.

Where your mother may have told you that breakfast was the most important meal of the day, new research is finding that skipping meals — going longer between meals — can actually extend life spans.

Studies done recently by the NIA have found that intermittent fasting — even eating every other day — can lower the risk of developing such age-related diseases as Parkinson's disease, Alzheimer's disease and strokes.

The studies also indicate that, beyond benefits to the brain, fasting protects animals from developing diabetes by helping cells metabolize glucose and it also helps the cardiovascular system.

Dr. Mark Mattson, director of neuroscience research at the NIA, says fasting seems to help the body's ability to handle stress — just as exercise does. "In our studies, though, intermittent fasting was even more effective than exercise at lowering heart rate and blood pressure."

Why? One theory of fasting holds that our bodies evolved in a feast-or-famine world where we ate woolly mammoth one day and went hungry the next. Today, most of us can pig out all day long if we wish, but that keeps our blood sugar at an extreme level. The blood sugar must be metabolized, which creates oxidation — which in turn creates the free radicals that modern theory holds are doing us in.

Eating three or more meals a day also gives our cells a steady supply of glucose, which makes the cells resistant to insulin, the hormone that transports glucose from our blood into cells. Insulin resistance in another word is diabetes.

"Intermittent fasting changes all that," Mattson told *Health* magazine. He says fasting causes brain cells to ready themselves with proteins, which tell individual cells to shut down until the stress is gone. And fasting also prompted the brain to generate new cells in case the stress of not eating causes some to die off. And in the body as a whole, the ability of cells to accept insulin is raised as cells poise themselves to glean whatever nutrition may come along.

A study of overweight diabetics proved this. One half of the group of 54 persons ate a standard low-calorie diet, while the others periodically cut back to 500 calories for one day. At the end of the 20-week study, glucose metabolism was improved in the group that cut back in calories from time to time.

The point, though, is not about weight loss. In an NIA study done on mice, the overall caloric intake was the same between those that fasted and those that didn't. And researchers caution that some diabetics being treated with drugs that keep blood sugar at low levels could find fasting risky, because their blood sugar could fall to dangerous levels.

But, says Dr. Mattson, people who are eating healthfully should be able to skip a meal here and there and get the benefits occasional fasting seems to provide. "If you're otherwise healthy, skipping a meal or even two now and then won't hurt you," he says, "assuming that your diet is a pretty healthy one."

And what of the great low-carbohydrate diet debate?

It remains a great debate.

A study in the *New England Journal of Medicine* found recently that forgetting the carbs and sticking with protein and fatty foods will make you lose more weight than a simple low-calorie diet in the short term, or six months. But the study found that the difference in weight lost between the two diets was insignificant after one year.

Proponents of low-carb diets such as the famous Atkins Diet claim that such a diet is the most natural for us, as humans only in the past 10,000 years — or since the domestication of grains — have eaten grains, cereals, starches and processed sugars in abundance. Proponents also say a diet high in protein and dairy products also helps control blood sugar better and reduce insulin levels, which in turn causes the body to burn its stored fat for energy.

And one study, done way back in 1965, showed that a high-fat, low-carbohydrate diet of 1,000 calories a day resulted in a greater weight loss over 10 days than did fasting. Also, despite the high-fat intake in a low-carb diet such as Atkins, low-carb dieters in one study had "significantly greater" improvements in levels of triglycerides and HDL cholesterol — the "good" cholesterol.

But critics point to a low amount of dietary fiber, which can lead to chronic bowel disease and constipation, and also say that the metabolic processes used to convert fat to energy in our bodies can lead to a buildup of uric acid, as well as a metabolic state called ketosis, which can cause headaches, nausea, fatigue, dehydration and dizziness.

As mentioned, the sides have squared off, while nutritionists and researchers continue to try to get to the bottom of the low-carb issue. As one commentator put it: "Those who have difficulty accepting the notion that loading up on fatty foods could be good for you can take comfort in the fact that the final word is not yet in."

CHAPTER 6

Heart Attack and Vine

While debate rages on and on and on in some areas of nutrition research, the results on other foods and their health-giving properties have been in for millennia.

For instance, fruit = good.

Especially, researchers are finding, fruits with deeply colored flesh — fruits such as plums, watermelon and even pomegranates.

The lycopene that makes tomatoes red and the anthocyanins that give blueberries and strawberries their deep hues have been associated with special health-giving effects.

One study published in the *Journal of Clinical Nutrition* found great benefits deriving from one of those deep-red fruits — the pomegranate. The study found that just 2 ounces of pomegranate juice daily had a 9 percent boost in the levels of their bodies' antioxidants. "Our belief is that if you drink 6 ounces daily, this protection increases," says Dr. Harley Liker, assistant clinical professor of medicine at the University of California-Los Angeles School of Medicine.

Researchers at Technion-Israel Institute in Israel also found that pomegranate juice may help slow aging and also protect the body against heart disease. "Pomegranate juice is the most potent antioxidant among all of the juices studied," said Dr. Michael Aviram, who has studied its properties. "It's extremely beneficial in preventing arteriosclerosis, or hardening of the arteries."

The buildup of plaque — potential blockages — was reduced 44 percent in mice given pomegranate juice, according to one study. Dr. Liker said the fruit can inhibit the oxidation of low-density cholesterol.

"This is the second way pomegranate juice helps your heart," Dr. Liker said. "It helps reduce plaque accumulation, which can cause heart disease. We also found that there's a third way pomegranate juice boosts cardio-vascular health. There is recent evidence that the juice inhibits platelet aggregation, or the grouping of blood platelets, that can cause serious strokes."

The juice can also lower blood pressure. "It works by blocking the ACE enzyme, much like prescription pills do, but in a much more natural way," Dr. Liker said. "Some studies have shown that pomegran-ate juice inhibits ACE enzymes by a signif-icant 36 percent."

Blueberries also have been found to be rich in antioxidants and other health-giving com-pounds. In fact, one study found them to hold the most antioxidants among berries.

Research on rats has found that blueberries helped their coordination and mental acuity — and did better even than those rats fed strawberries and spinach, which have also been touted as improving mental abilities.

The rats in one study, which were the human equivalent of being in their 60s, were fed blueberry extract for two months — which according to their rate of aging made them in their mid-70s at the study's end. "The blueberry-fed rats did better on standard rat tests, like swimming in a water maze or finding an underwater platform in murky water," the study said. "But they also did better on tests involving a spinning rod or an inclined rod — good tests of coordination."

What in the blueberries was responsible for these anti-aging phenomena? Researchers theorize that much of the improvement in the older rats' coordination could be owed to the antioxidants in the blueberries, which may have repaired the damage from oxidation and the scouring of free radicals in the rats' brains.

"Diets rich in fruits and vegetables have been shown to reduce the risk of heart disease and cancer," the study's authors noted. "The rats ate supplements made from blueberry juice, but the researchers think the whole fruit may confer even more benefits. You can't overdose on blueberries."

Researchers at the U.S. Department of Agriculture Human Nutrition Center have ranked blueberries at the top of a list of 40 other fruits and vegetables.

"Blueberries are associated with numerous health benefits including protection against urinary tract infections, cancer, age-related health conditions and brain damage from strokes," noted one writer. "They may also reduce the buildup of so-called 'bad' cholesterol, which contributes to heart disease and stroke."

The European blueberry, known as the bilberry, has been shown to prevent and even reverse macular degeneration, a common cause of blindness in the elderly.

Other berries have similar properties, though none ranks as high as blueberries in health-giving and even health-restoring properties. Cranberries also have been shown to protect against cancer, stroke and heart disease. The berries are loaded with polyphenols, which are potent antioxidants — and research has found cranberries may prevent the growth of human breast-cancer cells, as well as prevent gum disease and help heal stomach ulcers.

Experts advise persons to chew cranberries whole to get their entire health benefits. Sun-dried cranberries are also a good way to go — they retain much more of their sugar and are not as tart as their fresh counterparts.

Other berries have been proven to have heavy antioxidant concentrations. Strawberries, for instance, come in second only to blueberries in oxidants. They also have more vitamin C than any other berry.

Strawberries also contain the antioxidants anthocyanin and ellagic acid, which have been shown to fight the development of cancer. And studies have shown promise in fighting the development of heart disease.

Likewise, raspberries have cancer-fighting phytochemicals and also contain calcium, folic acid, fiber and vitamins A, C and E. They also have been found to provide protection from esophageal and other cancers.

And that longtime favorite summertime treat, watermelon, is known to be full of lycopene, which is a powerful antioxidant in its own right. Lycopene has been shown to improve the circulation of blood and can also prevent or reduce wrinkles in the skin.

Watermelon also has vitamins A, B6, C and thiamin.

Grape seeds have proved to be one of the most abundant sources of antioxidants, as well. In fact, grape-seed extract is more powerful as an antioxidant than vitamins C or E.

In a study at Creighton University, grape-seed extract was compared to the effectiveness of vitamins E and C in ridding the body of free radicals. The grape-seed acid KO'd 81 percent of the free radicals, compared to 44 percent being neutralized by vitamin E and just 19 percent being stymied by vitamin C.

Grape-seed extract was also found in a French study to lower the levels of bad cholesterol — LDLs — while raising the level of antioxidant enzymes by 67 percent.

What's more, grape-seed extract has proven cancer-fighting abilities — at least in laboratory animals. A University of Illinois study found grape-seed extract reduced tumors in lab animals by 88 percent. When applied to skin, the extract inhibited tumor growth by 78 percent — and also reduced cancerous cells in the breast, lung and stomach by 47 percent.

On to veggies! And our mantra: Eat your veggies. Eat your veggies.

Why? All right, we already said it. But we'll say it again.

Veggies are mainstays of your health — and can even help you live longer.

One study, done at Loma Linda University in California, found that a person who is a vegetarian for 20 years or more can expect to add four years to their lives.

"We are the first to come up with a life-expectancy figure showing a very important increase in life expectancy for those who follow a vegetarian diet for a long period of time," said the study's leader, Dr. Pramil Singh.

The study looked at 7,100 adherents to the Adventist religion who had been monitored for more than 40 years. Because of exact data which tracked the group over time, the study was able to isolate those who had been vegetarians and lapsed, as well as those who stuck to the church principles promoting vegetarianism — "enough people with which to make mortality comparisons," said Dr. Singh.

"Survival data indicate that long-term

vegetarians do experience a significant 3.6-year survival advantage over short-term vegetarians," Dr. Singh related. On average, those who had been vegetarians for more than 20 years lived to 86.5 years, while those who lapsed had an average life span of 82.9 years.

Other studies have shown similar results. When meat shortages during World War II left Scandinavians protein-challenged and reliant on vegetables, there was a noticeable drop in the mortality rate. After the war, a higher mortality rate returned with supplies of meat.

Another study found that, when compared to mortality expectations drawn from the population at large, vegetarians had a lower mortality rate than did non-vegetarians. The lowest mortality was found in cardiovascular diseases and deaths from cancer were one-half the overall rate in men and three-quarters of the overall rate in women. The study also found a reduction in ischemic heart diseases — strokes.

"When the strict and moderate vegetarians were analyzed separately, the strongest differential was found for ischemic heart diseases, which were much less frequent among strict vegetarians for both sexes," the study reported. "Some non-dietary factors, such as higher socioeconomic status, virtual absence of smoking and lower body mass index, may also have contributed to the lower mortality of the study participants."

That last part may be the key to the study group's overall better longevity than the vegetarianism itself. Other studies have not been as conclusive — some, in fact, have shown no difference in mortality between vegetarians and non-vegetarians.

The difference may be in the lifestyle.

The Adventists noted in the study above did more than eat their spinach: 40 percent of them exercised "vigorously" — there's that word again — for at least 15 minutes three times a week and fewer than 1 percent of them smoked. The researchers estimated that those two factors — exercise and not smoking — could account for as much as 10 extra years of life in the Adventist population.

The Adventists' rate of vegetarianism was significantly higher than the U.S. population as a whole — but so was their rate of exercise. So was their good health a result of veggies or exercise?

Said Dr. Susan Jebb, head of nutrition research at Britain's Medical Research Council's human-nutrition research unit: "It may well be a little bit of each."

Still, it seems safe to say that a person who is a vegetarian also is a person who cares more about their health. Getting regular exercise, not smoking and eating nutritious food seems to go hand-in-hand with vegetarianism, so it's impossible to isolate one factor as being responsible for better health.

CHAPTER 7

The Right Stuff

Yes, Ma, we know, you don't have to shout: We should be eating enough fruits and vegetables and plant-based foods to ensure we get the right amount of minerals and vitamins each and every day.

Well, the fact remains that, by and large, we aren't.

In fact, there are many reasons we may

not be getting the right amounts of vitamins and minerals.

People who are ages 70 or older, especially, are at risk of not getting the daily doses of vitamins they need to ward off disease.

"As you get older, health problems can contribute to a poor diet, making it difficult for you to get the vitamins and minerals you need," notes the Food and Nutrition Center at the renowned Mayo Clinic. "In addition, as you get older, your body may not be able to absorb vitamins B6, B12 and D like it used to, making supplementation more necessary. There is also evidence that a multivitamin may improve your immune function and decrease your risk for some infections when you're older."

The Mayo Clinic notes other situations where vitamin and mineral supplementation may be warranted:

- *If you're a postmenopausal woman.*
- *If you don't eat well.*
- *If you're on a low-calorie diet.*
- *If you smoke.*
- *If you drink excessively.*
- *If you're pregnant or trying to become pregnant.*

● *If, because of allergies or intolerance to certain foods, you eat a special diet.*
● *If your body can't absorb nutrients properly.*

There are indications that vitamin and mineral supplements are beneficial and not harmful at levels that at least match the Regular Dietary Allowances determined by the Food and Nutrition Board of the Institute of Medicine, part of the National Academy of Sciences. Daily Values are set by the Food and Drug Administration and are listed on the labels of vitamin and mineral supplements.

The International Longevity Center-USA notes: "Dietary deficiencies are a well-known risk factor for many diseases, including age-related diseases, such as cancer, cardiovascular disease and osteoporosis.

"Epidemiological data," the center continues, "on dietary intakes indicate that in persons whose diet is rich in fruits and vegetables, the risk of a variety of cancers is lowered by one-half ... research has indicated that supplementation can reduce the risk of age-related disease.

"For example, high levels of folate and vitamin B6 have recently been shown to reduce the risk of heart disease in women. Vitamin C has been particularly implicated in the reduction of smoking-induced oxidative damage, whereas vitamin E supplementation has been shown to reduce the risk of cancer and cardiovascular disease."

However, the ILC-USA says, "Most experts agree that including generous amounts of fruits and vegetables in the diet is preferred over dietary supplementation. Current recommendations are to include at least five servings of fruits and vegetables per day in the diet. A less desirable alternative is to recommend a multivitamin pill to the public in general. There is no evidence that this would be harmful and it is an inexpensive (5 to 10 cents/day/person) and simple approach."

But supplementation can't hurt — and may certainly help if you're not eating the right diet or have a condition or conditions that prevent you from using vitamins and minerals in your diet effectively. However, if you do choose to supplement vitamins and minerals, experts say you should not exceed 100 percent of the Daily Value listed on the bottle. Those values are:

Vitamin A	5,000 International Units (IU)
Vitamin C	60 milligrams (mg)
Vitamin D	400 IU
Vitamin E	20 IU (natural source)
	30 IU (supplemental source)
Vitamin K	80 micrograms (mcg)
Thiamin	1.5 mg
Riboflavin	1.7 mg
Niacin	20 mg
Pantothenic acid	10 mg
Pyridoxine	2 mg
Folic acid/folate	400 mcg
Vitamin B12	6 mcg
Biotin	300 mcg
Calcium	1,000 mg
Chloride	3,400 mg
Chromium	120 mcg
Copper	2 mg
Iodine	150 mcg
Iron	18 mg
Magnesium	400 mg
Manganese	2 mg
Molybdenum	75 mcg
Phosphorus	1,000 mcg
Potassium	3,500 mg
Selenium	70 mcg
Zinc	15 mg

A multivitamin, as mentioned above, can in many instances provide 100 percent or more of the Daily Value recommended. The percentage of Daily Value for all vitamins and minerals are listed on the bottle.

But keep in mind that some experts believe that individual RDAs vary from person to person based upon age, metabolism and other factors. Dr. Earl Mindell, author of *Earl Mindell's NEW Vitamin Bible*, in particular advises people to start with a good multivitamin as a base and add other vitamins and minerals according to specific health needs.

"Not everyone has the same metabolism and not everyone requires the same vitamins," says Dr. Mindell. "Everyone should take an all-natural, high-potency multiple vitamin/mineral complex for optimum health and optimal nutrition," he said.

"It should contain no artificial preservatives, colors or dyes and include digestive enzymes for better absorption. Make sure it contains a broad spectrum antioxidant formula that includes mixed carotenoids, lycopene, vitamins C and E and coenzyme-Q10," he recommended.

"A good multiple vitamin/mineral complex is the foundation and then you add layers of other vitamins as you need them," explained Dr. Mindell, author of numerous books on vitamins, health and nutrition.

In addition, men, women, children and people with special medical conditions should add the following vitamins to their daily routine:

WOMEN

In addition to the daily multiple vitamin and mineral complex with antioxidants, women should add:

Women 19-50: 500 mg of calcium and 250 mg of magnesium twice daily for a total of 1,000 mg of calcium and 500 mg of magnesium.

Women 50+: Vitamin E 400 IU (dry form) as well as 500 mg calcium and 250 mg magnesium, two tablets in the morning and at bedtime.

MEN

In addition to the daily multiple vitamin and mineral complex with antioxidants, men should add:

Men 19-30: 15 mg of zinc daily.

Men 30-50: 15-50 mg zinc, arginine time release, two tablets in the morning and two tablets in the afternoon.

Men 50+: 500 mg of glycinated calcium complex plus 25 mg of magnesium daily.

Also, certain conditions can be ameliorated with supplements, according to Dr. Mindell. Here's a sampling of vitamins that can help with certain ailments:

Arthritis. Extra vitamin C is a must if you suffer from this painful chronic condition, especially if you take lots of aspirin, which depletes vitamin C. 500 mg of vitamin C one to two times daily is helpful, says Dr. Mindell. Pantothenic acid (vitamin B5) in doses of 100 mg taken three times a day is a good idea as well.

Osteoporosis. Along with weight-bearing exercises that build bone density, Dr. Mindell recommends the following supplements: 1,000 mg of vitamin C with bioflavonoids, 400 IU of vitamin D, 400 to 800 IU of vitamin E in dry form, 100 to 200 mcg of vitamin K as well as 500 mcg of vitamin B12 in sublingual form daily.

Alzheimer's disease. In addition to the multiple vitamin and mineral complex containing major antioxidants and plenty of vitamin E, Dr. Mindell recommends taking choline.

Choline, a member of the B-complex can aid in the treatment of Alzheimer's. Dr. Mindell recommends taking one to five grams a day to help conquer the problem of memory loss, one of the symptoms of the disease.

Other recommended members of the B-complex that can aid memory loss: three mg of vitamin B1 (thiamin), 200 mcg of folacin and 25 mg of pantothenic acid.

Heart disease. With any heart condition you should be under a doctor's care, advises Dr. Mindell. Though the following supplements have been found to be safe and helpful, you should check with your physician to be sure they are not contraindicated. Take supplements of B6, B12 and folic acid, as well as vitamins C and E, recommends Dr. Mindell.

Dr. Mindell cautions that if you fall under more than one category, adjust accordingly so that you are not double-dosing yourself. Use common sense.

And be aware that dietary supplements, as pushed on the Internet, in stores, in books and in magazines reflect a multibillion-dollar industry at work. "Some people in the marketing industry are doing a good job of convincing older people that they need expensive nutritional supplements, some of which haven't been shown to be helpful or safe and some of which most older people may not even need," notes the National Institute on Aging. "Some of these claims give older adults the impression that certain supplements can restore youthful energy and strength.

"Buyer, beware — and check with your doctor before spending your hard-earned money on supplements that promise to restore youthful energy and strength."

And the International Longevity Center-USA notes: "Vitamin and mineral dietary supplements are considered safe for the general population when taken in doses that don't exceed the recommended dietary allowances. Some vitamins and minerals are toxic in high doses ... When in doubt, follow the RDA."

The ILC-USA also advises people to ask themselves the following questions when considering a dietary supplement:

- *Do you know if the substance has side effects?*
- *Do you know how the substance will react with drugs you are already taking?*
- *Do you know if you have a medical condition or health risk factor that makes it inadvisable for you to take the substance?*
- *Do you know if the substance is pure? Are you sure it doesn't contain other substances that may be harmful to your health?*
- *Do you know if you're taking the right dose?*

The NIA sounds a similar alarm in regard to over-the-counter supplements:

"Dietary supplements are now sold in almost every shopping mall, grocery store, drug store and convenience store, as well as on the Web. Each year people spend billions of dollars on these vitamins, minerals, herbs and hormones. They are hoping for more energy, stronger muscles, better memory, protection from disease and maybe even a longer life. The Food and Drug Administration ... does not oversee most of these products. So you can't be sure that a supplement's health claims are true or that they are safe to take for a long period of time ...

"Check with your doctor before buying pills or anything else that promises to do such things or to make a big change in the way you look or feel. These purchases may be unsafe or a waste of money. They might even interfere with other treatments."

And if you're wary about vitamin-and-mineral or other supplements anyway, there are ways to get more of the essential vitamins and minerals you need simply by eating the right foods, according to experts:

Calcium: Needed for strong bones and teeth, calcium can be found in milk, yogurt, ice cream, cheese, kale, collard greens and soybeans.

Copper: In addition to helping in the formation of red blood cells and maintaining the immune system, copper also promotes healthy nerves, bones and blood vessels. Copper can be obtained naturally though shellfish, whole grains, beans, nuts, potatoes, leafy green vegetables and prunes.

Iron: Essential for healthy red blood cells, iron can be found in liver, pork loin, oysters and clams, sardines and raisin bran cereal. It's also found, of course, in leafy green vegetables such as spinach, broccoli and lima beans.

Magnesium: Deficiencies in magnesium can cause abnormal heart rhythms. Get it from bran cereal, wheat germ, spinach, tofu, cooked beans and mixed nuts.

Manganese: Critical to cardiovascular health, the mineral can be obtained by eating nuts, wheat germ, oatmeal, pineapple and beans.

Potassium: Essential to proper heart function, potassium can be found in bananas, melons, prunes, turkey, fish, carrots and celery.

Zinc: Zinc has of late become a popular mineral for battling the common cold and is also touted as a stress-buster. The best sources for zinc are whole grains, beans and vegetables.

Again: If you have a condition which prevents you from absorbing and utilizing certain vitamins and/or minerals, you may need a daily supplement. Otherwise, many experts pooh-pooh the supposed health and longevity claims made by many supplements and recommend you get needed daily vitamins and minerals from a balanced, nutritious diet. And, as Dr. Mindell advises, a multivitamin a day is essential.

And your mom also wanted us to mention one more thing ...

Eat your fruits and vegetables!

CHAPTER 8

Doctor, Doctor

Of course eating, sweating, drinking and all of those other verbs are only half of the battle for maintaining good health. Regular check-ups are also part and parcel to being healthy.

Choosing the right doctor can also make a huge difference.

Though many insurance plans limit your choices in finding a primary-care physician — the doctor who will handle your overall health and, if needed, make referrals to other specialists for particular problems — you may have your choice of a doctor within the medical group named by your insurance company.

If you're limited by a particular insurance plan and have had recommendations for a certain doctor you think you'd want to handle your health matters, you'll still need to check with your insurance carrier to make sure your treatment by that physician is covered by your insurance.

What should you look for in a personal physician?

"In general, you want a doctor who is well-trained and competent," says one expert source. "You also want a doctor who cares about you, who will listen carefully to your concerns, who can explain things clearly and fully, and who can anticipate your health problems."

Depending upon your situation, you will probably make your choice of doctor from these three categories:

● **Family practitioner.** Family practitioners provide health care to all members of a family, no matter the age.

● **Internists.** An internist is a doctor for

adults and usually has training in an area of specialty, such as cardiology.

● **Geriatricians.** Geriatricians train in the area of family practice or internal medicine and then specialize in the care of older adults.

Once you've decided what type of doctor may be the best to handle your health care, call those offices and question the office staff about the doctors' education and training, the policies for payment and office procedure for appointments and emergency care.

You can also do some research on your own. Directories of medical providers may be found at your local library and there are Web sites that can give you information about specific credentials. You may want to check to see if your preferred doctor or doctors are board-certified, that is, that they've taken further training in a specific area of medicine beyond medical school. Doctors can become board-certified in numerous areas, including the primary-care fields of family practice, internal medicine and geriatrics.

Also, you can check with your local

county clerk's office to see if your prospective physician has been sued for malpractice.

"Please keep in mind," cautions one source, "that anyone can file a lawsuit at any time. The existence of a suit does not automatically indicate a physician practices medicine badly; it may mean that a patient was unhappy about the outcome of treatment received, possibly without fault of the physician. However, a pattern of legal actions may be cause for concern."

Once you've narrowed your list of prospective doctors, experts advise prospective patients to then make "get-acquainted" appointments with one or more physicians who seem like good fits with your needs. Make a list of your concerns and questions and, at those appointments, tell the doctors about your past medical and lifestyle history. It's important to be honest and at the same time not be shy about questioning the doctors about their practices.

"You'll probably have to pay for that appointment to come and sit and meet them," says one expert. "But if you choose to do that, it may give you helpful information. You may find that there's good rapport

— or that there's not — with the particular physician."

After the first meeting or meetings with the prospective doctors, experts advise you to ask yourself these questions:

Was I treated courteously?

Did the doctor answer all of my questions?

Was I rushed or dismissed?

If you did not feel a rapport from the doctor, or feel comfortable in placing your health care in his or her hands, move on to the next person on your list.

Once you have found a doctor who seems to meet the above criteria — one who takes time to listen, who truly seems interested in your care and who is an unquestionably proficient physician — you need to keep in mind that your health care is a two-way street. "A good doctor/patient relationship is a partnership, with both you and your doctor working together to solve your medical problems and maintain your good health," says one expert source. "Make sure that you feel comfortable working with your doctor."

CHAPTER 9

Let's Get Physical

Denial isn't a river in Egypt.

Denial courses through every human heart — and when it comes to maintaining good health, denial can become a risk factor in and of itself.

How many people do you know who are afraid to go to the doctor not because they're afraid to be poked and prodded and inspected like some prized heifer at the county fair, but because their doctors might actually find something wrong with them?

Instead, they follow an ignorance-is-bliss approach to their own bodies, avoiding that dreaded visit to the doctor until something — a bump, a flutter, an ache that won't go away — forces them out of denial and into sheer panic and foreboding. At that moment, they pick up the phone with trembling hands and arrange to be poked and prodded and inspected — and while usually their worst fears aren't borne out, on occasion there's bad news, along with those terrible words *if only we'd caught this sooner* ...

The fact is, when it comes to your health, you need to catch it while you can.

All health experts advise regular checkups and screenings, especially once people have crossed that bridge into their 40s. Because of all the accrual of trouble mentioned in Chapter 2 — those pesky radicals, cheeseburger sludge, old wounds, elusive time itself — bad things start happening to good people — as well as bad people — once they hit their 40s.

"As you get older, you get an increasing

risk for a number of chronic diseases," notes Dr. Edward Schneider, dean of the Leonard Davis School of Gerontology at the University of Southern California. "In fact, your risk increases exponentially for about a dozen diseases with each decade."

Incidences of heart disease, many cancers, osteoarthritis, Alzheimer's disease and diabetes, for example, increase dramatically past age 40, experts say.

The good news is that early detection remains one of the best methods of curing or stabilizing the effects of these diseases. You can stick your head in the sand and hope you won't get any or all of the above — or you can be proactive, and smart, and catch it while you can, before a particular disease or condition has progressed beyond the point where there's a real chance to treat it.

Simply put, if you're age 40 or older, one of the best things you can do right now to safeguard your health is to get regular checkups and screenings as suggested by your doctor. And just to get some idea of where the risk areas lay is a checklist of screenings for both men and women — what each does and how often you should have each done:

WOMEN

Breast cancer screening

Procedure	Purpose	Start age	How often
Mammogram	Detects cancer	40	Annually
Doctor's breast exam	Can detect tumors missed by mammography	20	Every three years for women 20-40; annually thereafter

Cervical cancer screening

Procedure	Purpose	Start age	How often
Pap smear and pelvic exam	Checks for cancer	18 or once a woman is sexually active	Annually; every 2-3 years after three normal tests in a row
Pap smear plus HPV DNA test & pelvic exam	More precise means to check for cancer	30	Every three years

Colorectal cancer screening

Procedure	Purpose	Start age	How often
Colonoscopy	Outpatient	50	Every 10

	procedure in which a long flexible instrument is inserted into the rectum to view the rectum and entire colon; considered by many experts to be the best screening for colon cancer		years or more frequently if there's a family history of colon cancer
Fecal occult blood test	Tests for blood in the stool, which can indicate cancer	50	Every five years
Flexible sigmoidoscopy	Outpatient test examines lower part of the large intestine	50	Every five years
Air-contrast barium enema	Reveals through X-ray any irregularities in the colon; is interchangeable with flexible sigmoidoscopy	50	Every five years

Skin cancer screening

Procedure	Purpose	Start age	How often
Total body skin exam	To detect precancerous and cancerous growths	50	Annually

Heart disease screening

Procedure	Purpose	Start age	How often
Blood cholesterol test	Measure total "good" and "bad" cholesterol as well as other blood fats	20	Every five years or as ordered by your doctor
Blood pressure check	Measures pressure, an indicator of risk of heart disease	18	At least every other year or more often if above normal
Fasting plasma glucose	Measures blood sugar	45	Every three years or as ordered by your doctor

Eye disease screening

Procedure	Purpose	Start age	How often
Glaucoma test	Measures eye pressure and eye health	60 for normal, healthy adults; 40 for those with family risk factors	Annually

Bone health

Procedure	Purpose	Start age	How often
Bone mineral density test	Is an indicator of bone strength and osteoporosis risk	65 or at menopause; earlier for women who have fragility or other factors	Ask your doctor

Thyroid health

Procedure	Purpose	Start age	How often
Thyroid hormone test	Blood test checks whether thyroid gland is working properly	35	Every five years

Vaccines/immunizations

Procedure	Purpose	Start age	How often
Tetanus booster	Restore protection against tetanus	Varies	Every 10 years
Pneumonia vaccine	Gives lifelong protection from pneumonia	20	65; earlier for those with risk factors of lung disease, heart failure or alcoholism
Influenza vaccine	Provides protection from common influenza strains	50 or earlier	Annually

MEN

Prostate cancer screening

Procedure	Purpose	Start age	How often
Digital rectal exam	Checks for telltale lumps or other abnormalities	50; 40-45 for men at risk	Annually

Procedure	Purpose	Start age	How often
Prostate-specific antigen blood test	Blood test to screen for high PSA levels, which could be a sign of inflammation or cancer	50; 40-45 for men at risk	Annually

Colorectal cancer screening

Procedure	Purpose	Start age	How often
Colonoscopy	Outpatient procedure in which a long flexible instrument is inserted into the rectum to view the rectum and entire colon; considered by many experts to be the best screening for colon cancer	50	Every 10 years or more frequently if there's a family history of colon cancer
Fecal occult blood test	Tests for blood in the stool, which can indicate cancer	50	Every five years

Flexible sigmoidoscopy	Outpatient test examines lower part of the large intestine	50	Every five years
Air-contrast barium enema	Reveals through X-ray any irregularities in the colon; is interchangeable with flexible sigmoidoscopy	50	Every five years

Skin cancer screening

Procedure	*Purpose*	*Start age*	*How often*
Total body skin exam	To detect precancerous and cancerous growths	50	Annually

Heart disease screening

Procedure	*Purpose*	*Start age*	*How often*
Blood cholesterol test	Measure total "good" and "bad" cholesterol as well as other blood fats	20	Every five years or as ordered by your doctor

Blood pressure check	Measures pressure, an indicator of risk of heart disease	18	At least every other year or more often if above normal
Fasting plasma glucose	Measures blood sugar	45	Every three years or as ordered by your doctor

Eye disease screening

Procedure	Purpose	Start age	How often
Glaucoma test	Measures eye pressure and eye health	60 for normal, healthy adults; 40 for those with family risk factors	Annually

Thyroid health

Procedure	Purpose	Start age	How often
Thyroid hormone test	Blood test checks whether thyroid gland is working properly	35	Every five years

Vaccines/immunizations

Procedure	Purpose	Start age	How often
Tetanus booster	Restore protection against tetanus	Varies	Every 10 years
Pneumonia vaccine	Gives lifelong protection from pneumonia	20	65; earlier for those with risk factors of lung disease, heart failure or alcoholism
Influenza vaccine	Provides protection from common influenza strains	50 or earlier	Annually

The previous charts are rough guides to the ages at which and the frequency with which these screenings should be performed. They also may serve as minimums and you doctor may want to screen you more frequently if there are risk factors involved in your personal health or if you have a family history that indicates a predisposition for any disease or diseases.

You should provide your doctor with a detailed family history — incidences and age of onset of prostate cancer, breast cancer or other possibly hereditary trouble. Your doctor can then make a better judgment of how often to screen you and which areas of your health merit the most attention.

We're going to explore in more detail in the chapters ahead the major health concerns listed in the charts — and what you can do to protect and revitalize your health by making healthy lifestyle choices, as well as undergoing these screenings.

CHAPTER 10

Aging Ain't for Sissies

Colonoscopy. There. We said it — and we're glad.

Many people don't like that word, with its sinister associated images. But avoid the word, and the procedure itself, at your peril. Colorectal cancer, if left undetected, can be more sinister than you may know.

The facts: Colorectal cancer is the No. 2

killer in the United States. Ninety percent of people who get colorectal cancer are older than age 50. While the actual risk of developing cancer sometime in your lifetime is about 6 percent, or 1 in 17, experts advise several tests be done either every year or every five years, as mentioned in the charts. For those with a history of colorectal cancer in their families, those considered above-average for a risk of developing the cancer, the intensity of testing for the cancer increases.

Can colon cancer be prevented? Perhaps. Or at least the risk can be lowered by eating right, not smoking, not drinking alcohol to excess and by getting exercise.

"Some studies show a lower risk of colon cancer among those who are moderately active on a regular basis and more vigorous activity may even further reduce the risk of colon cancer," the American Cancer Society (ACS) notes. "Being inactive is linked more to an increased risk of cancer of the colon than cancer of the rectum. Diets high in vegetables may reduce the risk and diets high in red meat may increase the risk of colon cancer. Some evidence shows that folic acid supplements may reduce the risk of colon cancer.

"The best advice to reduce the risk of colon cancer," says the ACS, is to:

- *Increase your physical activity*
- *Eat more vegetables and fruit*
- *Limit intake of red meats*
- *Avoid obesity*
- *Avoid excess alcohol.*

Cancer of the colon and/or rectum comes in the form of a malignant tumor that arises on the wall of the large intestine. These tumors can spread to other parts of the body, such as the liver or lungs, making the disease particularly dangerous. Most cancers begin as a tiny clump of noncancerous, or benign, cells called polyps. If left, these polyps can turn malignant. If caught early enough, the five-year survival rate is 95 percent, said Dr. LaMar McGinnis, senior medical consultant to the American Cancer Society.

The National Polyp Study found that in 90 percent of people who had polyps removed, there was a 90 percent drop in the incidence of colon cancer. Because colon cancer can be slow growing, and it can take several years for polyps to turn cancerous, early detection is vital and usually successful in warding off malignancies.

There are many risk factors involved in the development of colorectal cancer — and many of them are the usual culprits when talking about maintaining good health. Smoking, excessive drinking, a sedentary lifestyle and obesity have all been implicated in colorectal cancer.

In addition, a personal history of inflammatory bowel disease and in some instances heredity — especially among Jews of Eastern European descent — can put you at an above-average risk for colorectal cancer. As mentioned above, a history of colon cancer or precancerous polyps also puts you more at risk to develop colorectal cancer. Talk to your doctor about any risk factors you may have to decide the best course of testing for colorectal cancer.

For those with what is considered average risk — in other words, there is no history in their family or other risk factors — screening is recommended to begin at age 50, according to the U.S. Multisociety Task Force on Colorectal Cancer. Those at normal risk are recommended to undergo either a fecal occult blood test annually or a flexible sigmoidoscopy every five years — or both.

The fecal occult blood tests (FOBTs) involve chemical tests on a sample of your stool to detect the presence of blood that otherwise can't be seen and which can indicate slow bleeding from a polyp or tumor in your intestine. The test can be done in your doctor's office, or done with a kit at home, and it is non-invasive. Because cancers sometimes bleed only intermittently, the test is generally done on three consecutive days to ensure no trouble lurks in your intestines. Those at average risk for colorectal cancer are urged to have an FOBT every year.

A more invasive procedure with the grim-sounding flexible sigmoidoscopy is recommended at age 50 and then at least every five years thereafter for people who are at average risk for colorectal cancer.

In this procedure, a flexible fiberoptic tube with a light at the tip is inserted into the anus and through it your doctor can view the rectum and the sigmoid colon — about the last two feet of your intestine. Air is also pumped into your bowel, inflating it for a better look-see, and there may be some feelings of cramping or an urge to have a bowel movement. The procedure usually takes just 15 minutes, unless polyps are found and biopsies need to be done.

"Approximately 50 percent of colorectal cancers and polyps are found to be within reach of a flexible sigmoidoscope," says one source. "The removed polyps are examined by a pathologist under a microscope to determine if the polyps are benign, malignant or precancerous."

If blood is detected during the FOBT or polyps found during the flexible sigmoidoscopy, your doctor will want to find the source of the bleeding by means of a colonoscopy. The colonoscopy remains the best way in which your doctor can examine the length of your colon to make sure no polyps, tumors or precancerous growths are lurking inside.

"The majority (greater than 90 percent) of the polyps detected at colonoscopy can be removed painlessly and safely during the colonoscopic examination," says one expert source. "Individuals with precancerous polyps have a higher than average risk for developing colon cancer and are advised to return for periodic surveillance colonoscopies."

No matter your risk for developing colorectal cancer, many doctors recommend colonoscopies, and not the less-invasive flexible sigmoidoscopy, beginning at age 50 and then every seven to 10 years thereafter if no polyps are found. This is because half of the cancers and polyps are found in the upper part of the colon, beyond the reach of the sigmoidoscopy.

Experts say that in the hands of an experienced practitioner, a colonoscopy is relatively painless. But it goes without saying that the procedure causes a lot of apprehension among patients by virtue of its invasiveness and because of the area of the body involved. For that reason, doctors will often prescribe a mild sedative and/or an opiate pain medication such as Demerol to reduce the anxiety.

Recent advances have led to one other test to detect cancers and polyps, and though the test is less invasive than a colonoscopy, it is also less reliable. Called a virtual colonoscopy, it is performed by means of a

CT scan. Following a full cleaning of your bowels, the test is done by inserting a tube into your anus and blowing air into your intestines. Doctors can then view a two-dimensional image of your intestines and a virtual image of your colon.

Other new advances also show promise. The 3-D virtual colonoscopy allows doctors to take images of the colon and analyze them for growths. A study published in the *New England Journal of Medicine* reported that 87.8 percent of colon polyps as small as 6 millimeters in diameter were identified with this technique — while 98.8 percent of polyps 10 millimeters or larger were also found. The test requires patients to fast prior to the test and also take a laxative to cleanse the colon. But no anesthesia is required and there are no tubes being inserted into the colon. Nor is there danger of perforation of the colon wall.

Unfortunately, the test cannot detect the tiny polyps a colonoscopy can find. It also can't remove any polyps that might be found — and keep in mind that polyps and tumors are found in 30 percent to 40 percent of people who have colonoscopies.

Two more tests, the air-contrast barium enema and the single-column barium enema, are in decline as doctors turn more and more to colonoscopies for full and accurate testing for colorectal cancer. If abnormalities are detected through one of these tests, you will still be a candidate for a colonoscopy for further examination of your intestines. And some doctors recommend that a flexible sigmoidoscopy be done in conjunction with a barium enema test.

The upshot?

The American Cancer Society recommends the following schedule of screenings after age 50 for men and women:

- *An annual fecal occult blood test*
- *A flexible sigmoidoscopy every five years*
- *A double-contrast barium enema every five years*
- *A colonoscopy every 10 years*

As with people who have a family history of colon cancer or polyps, people who have a personal history of chronic inflammatory bowel disease should also begin screening for colorectal cancer earlier than age 50, says the ACS.

Some doctors insist that a colonoscopy is

the best method of detecting all colon cancers and polyps and thus preventing or treating colorectal cancer. One study of more than 3,000 people found abnormalities in 128 people. A flexible sigmoidoscopy done on these same 128 people missed polyps that were out of reach of the sigmoid scope.

Beyond the FOBTs, each test — barium enemas, the flexible sigmoidoscopy and the colonoscopy — each have their own levels of discomfort and preparation and colonoscopies carry a small risk of perforation of the colon, which can lead to hospitalization.

Because of this risk and because many people are indeed reluctant to go through the more invasive tests — with the fasting, the enemas, the sedation — doctors are looking for easier ways to detect colon cancer.

"People don't like to restrict their diets before a test and they hate the messiness of the test for blood in the stool," said the American Cancer Society's Dr. LaMar McGinnis. "They fear the embarrassment of the flexible sigmoidoscopy and conventional colonoscopy. As a consequence, only half of those who should be screened — everyone over age 50 — ever are. And tragically, only 37 percent of colorectal cancers are caught at the early stages."

Trying to find a way around the sigmoidoscopies and colonoscopies and get more people to be tested, researchers are investigating whether molecular "markers" can be employed to detect abnormalities in the colon. One test, called the COLARIS, is a blood test that can reveal the mutated MLH1 or MLH2 genes in your blood. These killer mutations are present in the blood of people who have a genetic predisposition to colon cancer — a predisposition that can raise the chances of developing colon cancer from 3 percent to a frightening 80 percent. But if these mutated genes can be identified early enough, doctors can monitor at-risk patients that much more closely and, if colon cancer is later detected, treat them in the earliest stages of the disease.

Another cutting-edge test, called the GCC-B1, can tell colon cancer survivors if their cancer has returned. The GCC-B1 had a 99 percent success rate in finding recurring colorectal cancers in a recent study.

Another noninvasive advance is a fecal test that detects cancer before there is even blood in the stool. It works by identifying tiny strands of DNA as well as mutated genes shed by colorectal cancerous cells, allowing doctors to diagnose the disease at its most curable stage.

But a colonoscopy is still the most successful way to find colon cancer. And there's no reason to be squeamish. With colorectal cancer the No. 2 cancer killer in the United States, screening for this deadly disease is essential. Consult with your doctor to determine which of the described tests are best for you. And remember — growing old ain't for sissies.

CHAPTER 11

Makin' Whoopee

That last chapter wasn't all that much fun, we know. So we thought we'd talk about something slightly less, er, clinical just for a minute.

Remember that well-worn part of the book *The Godfather* where Sonny's schtuppin' that gal against the door while Connie's wedding is swirling outside?

This is that part of our book.

It's about sex.

The act of sex, like most other aspects of our bodily functions, has been studied to death. And the news regarding health is all good.

One study of 35,000 people found that the sex act reduces the effects of negative emotions and stress — and in fact said not having sex can lead to premature death.

"A premature cessation of sexual intercourse in early old age has been found to be associated with an increased mortality risk," said the study's author. "Society assumes that the frequency and quality of sex declines with age. Sexuality is not the prerogative of younger people, nor should it be, although it is widely regarded as such. There is no fixed biological limit to a good sex life and people who have sex tend to be happier and have healthier cardiovascular systems."

And, if you're male, there's even more good news about sex.

Contradicting earlier studies of sexually active men, a new study has found that frequent ejaculation does not lead to a greater risk of prostate cancer — and in fact may prevent the disease.

Frequent sex for men "possibly could be associated with a lower risk of prostate cancer," said Dr. Michael Leitzmann, an epidemiologist at the National Cancer Institute and the author of the study.

The study looked at almost 30,000 doctors, dentists and other health professionals ranging in age from 46 to 81 who were asked how often they ejaculated, including masturbation and sexual intercourse.

Those who reported between four and seven ejaculations a month were 11 percent less likely to develop prostate cancer than those who ejaculated no more than three times a month. And each increase of three ejaculations per week over a man's lifetime correlated with another 15 percent drop in the risk of prostate cancer.

Men who ejaculated at least 21 times per month had 33 percent less chance of developing prostate cancer, according to the study, "suggesting that frequent ejaculation does indeed protect the prostate from growing tumors," one account of the study reported. "The researchers suggest that ejaculation could help purge the prostate of cancer-causing chemicals or stunt the formation of crystalloids that have been linked to tumors in some men."

Also, the relief of stress associated with ejaculation could prompt hormonal changes that affect the likelihood of the prostate undergoing cancerous changes, another theory holds.

Of course, at least in regard to men, sexual function and desires can change over time. "Beginning at age 40," notes *AltHealth*, "there is a definite decrease in sexual ability and libido. The older the man, after age 40, the more likely he is to experience erectile dysfunction.

"Damage to arteries, smooth muscles and fibrous tissues, often as a result of disease, is the most common cause of impotence. Diseases — including diabetes, kidney disease, chronic alcoholism, multiple sclerosis, atherosclerosis and vascular disease — account for about 70 percent of cases of impotence. Between 35 and 50 percent of men with diabetes experience impotence."

Not smoking, not drinking to excess, eating the right diet and getting plenty of vigorous exercise can help men not only maintain their cardiovascular health, but their ability to have sex. Women approaching or going through menopause may experience vaginal dryness and, thus, pain during sex. Experts recommend a vaginal lubricant to help avoid this problem.

Women, like men, "may notice a declining interest in sex during menopause," notes *AltHealth*. "It's a common side effect while the body is attempting to adjust. Estrogen replacement therapy (more on this later) can help return your libido to normal ... once the unpleasant side effects of menopause have stopped, the drive returns and could even be enhanced."

Indeed, one study at Duke University found that 13 percent of women have more interest in sex after menopause. The lack of sexual interest in older women, sex-research pioneers Masters and Johnson found, had more to do with an unstimulating relationship than other mental or physical factors.

Experts advise couples to be open and honest about their sex lives and to avail themselves of plenty of time for foreplay and also advise patience with each other as age changes the sexual equation. "Growing old brings about increasingly complex physical problems," notes one expert. "Coping with such problems requires a sexual partner who is not only willing to put up with some inconveniences but is also willing to communicate on an extremely intimate level to accommodate his or her partner's new sexual needs and limitations. Such pressures on the sexual relationship require a deep love and desire to stay with the sexual partner regardless of personal inconvenience.

"Every stage of life has sexual challenges and adjustments," notes the book *Sexual Survival in Perspective*. "Every stage has sexual casualties, but more are likely to occur as the years pass. Some couples become discouraged, lose their sexual relationship and give up physical contact with each other. For too many, marriage then evolves into a sibling-like living arrangement, with separate bedrooms. Sexual aging does not have to be like that. There is hope as long as you're willing to learn and experiment and keep a sense of humor. Sometimes sex can be even better than before because the quality of the relationship is more mature."

As well, "Older men feel more relaxed, tend to be more experienced and have better sexual control over the timing of their orgasms than young men do ... The older woman has sexual advantages, too, because she's more comfortable with her sexuality, usually has more insight into her sexual needs and may be able to express them to her husband. She may be more open to new sexual techniques and stimuli than she was when she was younger, revitalizing a boring sex life by exploring new levels of intimacy."

So have sex — it's good for the body and soul. Stay in shape. Don't smoke. Communicate with your spouse or significant other. A good sex life is a big part of our overall health after age 40.

CHAPTER 12

Your Cheatin' Heart

"Increasing age is one of the strongest risk factors we have for heart disease," says Dr. Lori Mosca, director of preventive cardiology at New York-Presbyterian Hospital. "It becomes a very common condition after the age of 50 or 60."

Experts have noted that heart functions slow with age. Muscle strength within the heart decreases, pumping power declines, and the maximal heart rate — the number of times your heart contracts in a minute — also slows. The result, as smaller amounts of blood are pumped to the heart, can be high blood pressure.

There's not much we do can about the effects of simple aging — those antioxidants bounding around the cell walls within heart and other muscles and tissues that have a negative effect over time. But we can keep our hearts healthier by avoiding the risk factors associated with high blood pressure, heart disease and other circulatory ailments.

"From age 40 through 70, the five major risk factors for heart disease are family history, smoking, high cholesterol, diabetes and high blood pressure," notes one expert medical source. "But apart from family history and smoking, the others are related to diet, weight and inactivity. Directly, age is not a risk factor, but people tend to put on weight and become more inactive as they age. And a combination of other factors, such as continuing heart-unhealthy habits and diets, takes its toll as people age and as such age is a risk factor for the other risk factors."

In other words, whatever you're doing, stop it. If you're not exercising, stop not exercising. Don't smoke. Eat healthier. You can delay the aging of your heart and arteries and be healthy — even after ages 40, 50, 60 or more — and delay or prevent the onset of atherosclerosis.

"Atherosclerosis, once thought to be an aging disorder, is now known to be a progressive narrowing of the arteries over time which is fed by rich diets high in cholesterol and fats and aggravated by smoking and high blood pressure," says one expert. Known as the "silent killer," coronary heart disease (CHD) can slip up on people who otherwise have no symptoms. Witness popular talk-show host David Letterman, who went in for a routine checkup several years ago and wound up being slapped to a gurney and sent into an immediate heart-bypass operation and a months-long recuperation.

Experts have developed a list of 23 risk factors for coronary heart disease, chief among them a history of cigarette smoking, high blood pressure, obesity, physical inactivity, diabetes and a family history of the disease.

One study recently added to a growing

body of evidence that body shape can also be a predictor of the disease.

Researchers from Wake Forest University Baptist Medical Center reported that the amount of fat in and around the abdominal organs is a good indicator of heart-attack risk in women. Women who are "apple" shaped, rather than "pear" shaped, were more likely to suffer heart attacks during the four-and-a-half years the study followed them. The researchers recommended that women diet and exercise to bring down their total weight.

"Coronary heart disease is the most common, chronic, life-threatening illness in the United States," says one expert source. "It affects 11 million Americans. Earlier in life, men have a greater risk of coronary heart disease than women. However, a woman's risk eventually equals or exceeds that of men after she begins menopause."

A buildup of fatty tissues inside the arteries that supply blood to the heart, also known as atherosclerosis, over time can constrict the coronary arteries, decreasing blood flow. The result can also be a blood clot in the arteries, which can lead to a heart attack.

"Symptoms of CHD usually develop insidiously," notes the Johns Hopkins University Health Disease Library. "In the early stages of the disease, there are generally no symptoms. As the disease progresses, angina (chest pain) may develop during periods of physical activity or emotional stress, because the narrowed arteries cannot supply the heart the increased amount of blood and oxygen necessary at those times. Angina usually subsides quickly with rest, but over time, symptoms arise with less exertion, and CHD may eventually lead to a heart attack. However, in a third of CHD cases, angina never develops and a heart attack can occur suddenly and with no prior warning."

Because of the stealth with which CHD can progress, experts advise regular testing to determine a person's risk of developing the disease. Depending on your risk factors — i.e., a history of smoking, inactivity, being overweight and/or a high-fat diet — these tests may include:

● **An EKG (electrocardiogram).** This fairly simple test can detect abnormalities in your heart rate and rhythm, which may suggest your heart isn't getting enough blood and oxygen.

● **Blood cholesterol tests.** These tests, which analyze the amounts of lipids, or fats, in your blood, can identify whether you are at risk to develop CHD. Doctors will analyze the amounts of so-called "good cholesterol" — also known as high-density lipids — and the amounts of "bad cholesterol," or low-density lipids.

● **Blood test for enzymes.** This simple blood test can tell whether certain enzymes are leaking from damaged heart-muscle cells into your bloodstream.

● **Exercise stress test.** Your doctor will have you walk on a treadmill and attached sensors will monitor blood pressure reactions.

● **Imaging test with radioactive tracers.** In this test, a radioactive material is sent into your bloodstream and courses through your heart muscle, allowing your doctor to monitor the working of your heart muscle.

● **Coronary angiogram.** Considered the most accurate way to measure the health of your arteries, the test involves the placing of a long, thin tube into an artery in the forearm or groin. It is then threaded through the coronary arteries and dye is injected to identify narrowed or blocked arteries. The test requires sedation.

Also, a new test known as multidetector CT scans of the heart is showing promise in detecting blockages in arteries without the invasiveness of an angiogram. In the procedure, which uses special CT detector machines, X-rays pass through the heart and are picked up by detectors that pass the information on to a computer, which constructs an image of the heart and arteries. The greater the number of detectors in the CT machine, the greater the resolution of the picture. The test can take as little as 15 minutes, compared with 45 minutes for an angiogram — not to mention the eight hours or so of recovery time from the anesthetic. Where patients who came into an emergency room complaining of chest pains would formerly be admitted to a hospital and monitored for 24 hours, and might ultimately need to undergo an angiogram for a good look at the heart and arteries, the multidetector CT scan of the heart can more quickly detect whether there is a blockage or blockages causing a heart attack.

But the procedure, though new, is already

controversial. Some critics of the multidetector CT scans worry that the tests will lead to unnecessary treatments for problems that don't exist.

"Some heart experts see trouble ahead," noted *The New York Times* in an article about the test. "For example, the scans identify narrowed coronary arteries in people with no symptoms of heart disease, like chest pains. Once a narrowing is detected, many doctors and most patients want to fix it, inserting a stent or doing bypass surgery — even though research shows such actions will not prevent heart attacks in such patients."

Trouble can arise where there would have been none before if a blockage is found and during treatment by implanting a stent — a tiny screen that keeps the artery open — a catheter accidentally separates the layers of the coronary artery or if a tiny piece of plaque from an artery is knocked loose and travels to the brain, causing a stroke, some experts say.

Of course, the best way to avoid having to deal with such complications is to avoid the development of narrowed arteries. Eating a low-fat diet and getting lots of exercise may, in the absence of a family history of the disease, prevent the arteries from clogging. And experts also recommend the following in reducing your likelihood of developing CHD:

- *Quit smoking*
- *Reduce your LDL ("bad") cholesterol*
- *Reduce high blood pressure*
- *Eat a healthy diet*
- *Lose weight*
- *Exercise*

If your doctor detects CHD through any of the above methods, you may be urged to undergo a lifestyle change — i.e., quit smoking, change your diet, begin a regular exercise program — or you may be a candidate for more dramatic drug therapy.

These drugs could include nitrates, such as nitroglycerin, which widen blood vessels and allow a greater flow of blood to the heart. Depending on your condition, beta-blockers may be prescribed. These drugs slow your heart rate, decreasing the load on your heart and decrease the force of heart muscle contractions.

Doctors also often prescribe people older than age 50 to take an aspirin every day, which can reduce the risk of a heart attack in people who have already had one. There are also medications which can lower LDLs and prevent built-up plaques in your artery walls from tearing or breaking off, which can cause heart attacks.

Doctors are also coming up with new ways to lower cholesterol, especially in people who have an inherited tendency to have elevated levels of LDLs. One new technique, called LDL aphaeresis, is a procedure by which the LDLs are actually filtered out of the bloodstream.

The two-hour procedure is done every two weeks and doctors say just one treatment can lower LDL levels 60 percent to 70 percent.

"We put a needle in one arm vein and run the blood through a series of filters to remove the LDL or 'bad' cholesterol, after which the blood is returned to the patient's other arm," said Dr. Mark Deeg, professor of medicine at the University of Indiana School of Medicine and director of its Vascular Health Program.

The technique is aimed at the million-and-a-half Americans who have trouble getting their LDL levels below the standard benchmark of 200 because they suffer from familial hypercholesterolemia, an inherited disorder that prevents people from getting rid of their LDL.

"Normally, LDL cholesterol is removed from the blood by the liver, but people who suffer from familial hypercholesterolemia can't get rid of their LDL — and the result can kill them," said Dr. Deeg.

More invasive therapy may be required if blockages are found. This could begin with balloon angioplasty, in which a catheter is threaded from the groin or forearm and into the blocked vessel. A balloon at the tip is then inflated slightly and a stent may be inserted at that point to keep the artery open and blood flowing.

And, as mentioned above, if you have one or more severe blockages that are life-threatening and not treatable by balloon angioplasty, you may be a candidate for bypass surgery, in which sections of the blocked artery or arteries are removed and replaced by a clean section or sections from elsewhere in your body.

But prevention of CHD, as with all other diseases and disorders, remains the best cure. One of the best ways to prevent CHD is to eat right and get plenty of exercise — beginning in youth or even middle age.

"People who work out seriously and continuously for most of a decade have been seen to cut their age-related decline of a maximal heart rate in half," says one medical source. "So maintaining a healthy diet and regular activity level, and stopping unhealthy habits like smoking, go a long way in controlling heart-related problems."

One study found that cardio-respiratory fitness in early adulthood can decrease the chances of developing high blood pressure and diabetes.

"Americans need to become physically active early in life and continue to be active as they age in order to remain as healthy as possible," commented Dr. Barbara Alving, the acting director of the National Heart, Lung and Blood Institute.

But experts emphasized that physical activity can have health-giving benefits at any stage of life.

"Americans don't have to run marathons to improve their physical fitness," added Cheryl Nelson, the NHLBI project officer for the study. "They should try to engage in at least 30 minutes of a moderate-intensity physical activity such as brisk walking on most, and preferably all, days of the week. Being physically active will not only improve their fitness but also help them maintain a healthy weight, which in turn will protect their heart health."

You should also talk to your doctor about taking aspirin on a daily basis. Aspirin, which can interfere with your blood's clotting action, can reduce the clumping together of blood platelets. The U.S. Preventive Services Task Force, part of the Department of Health and Human Services, suggests taking a daily aspirin to keep your heart healthy if:

- *You're a man over 40 years old*
- *You're a postmenopausal woman*
- *You're younger than 40 but have risk factors for cardiovascular disease, such as smoking, high blood pressure, high cholesterol or lack of exercise*

CHAPTER 13

Stand By Your Man

Men, meet your prostate.

Helloooo, prostate.

What is the prostate? Well, Jimmy, it's a walnut-size gland that can create monster-size problems in men, especially when they're older than age 40.

But while prostate cancer is "the most frequent new cancer diagnosis in men," according to one source, and cancer of the prostate is second only to lung cancer as the leading cause of cancer in men, the good news is that several other maladies related to the prostate are not life-threatening and in fact are easily treatable.

So what the heck is the prostate? It's a gland whose main job is to produce fluid for semen. But as men age, and that role often diminishes, a common problem known as benign prostatic hyperplasia can develop — "one of the most common health problems faced by men over 40," according to one expert source. "In fact, about 50 percent of men will experience problems in their 60s, a number that grows to about 80 percent of men by the time they reach their 80s."

Simply put, benign prostatic hyperplasia (BPH) is an enlarged prostate. The good, and bad, news is that you're not to blame — unlike many illnesses and conditions in the medical annals, there's little reason to wish you'd done this or that in your younger days to avoid the problem now besting you in your middle-age years. It just happens, and experts are still unsure why, although there is some speculation that the growth is related to hormonal changes that occur later in life, especially increased levels of a hormone called DHT. But BPH, though a nuisance, is not life-threatening and is not related to cancer.

BPH does, however, cause discomfort. The prostate, located next to the urethra, from which urine is eliminated from the bladder, can begin to squeeze off the urethra as it grows, making it difficult to urinate. Urine remains in the bladder as it is unable to spill all of its contents — and this condition of blocked and irritated bladder can lead to more serious trouble, including infections and damage to the kidneys and bladder itself, if left untreated.

A weak urine stream, the need to urinate during the night, urgent urination, a burning sensation during urination, a stopping and starting of the urinary stream, and a sensation that the bladder is not emptying are all symptoms of BPH.

Your doctor can diagnose BPH by means of a digital rectal exam, a painless procedure in which the doctor feels inside the rectum to determine the size and consistency of the prostate. If BPH is suspected, you may be referred to a urologist for further tests, which can include an ultrasound examination, a urine flow study, an X-ray of the urinary tract, or a cytoscopy, in which a small viewing device is inserted through the urethra and bladder to get a good look at the prostate and any obstructions.

Treatment could include simply watching and waiting if you're not experiencing any symptoms or obstruction to the urinary flow. The treatment for BPH may also involve the use of drugs if your case is mild, but keep in mind that the drugs — such as Flomax, Proscar and Cardura — need to be taken for life to keep the symptoms of BPH at bay.

Your doctor may also recommend surgery if your symptoms are severe. These surgeries can remove excess prostate tissue and/or widen the neck of the urethra where it joins the bladder. While these surgeries can relieve symptoms, risks include impotence, incontinence and ejaculation problems.

New laser treatments, however, are lessening the invasiveness of treating BPH. These treatments can sometimes be performed on an outpatient basis, but "not all patients may benefit ... when surgery is needed," says one source.

Keep in mind, too, that a new treatment for BPH called ILC is showing "great promise" in treating the enlarged prostate. The procedure, which involves a fiber optic instrument, is minimally invasive and studies have shown it carries a lower or similar risk of side effects and postoperative complications when compared to normal surgery.

Also, experts say there are things you can do to either prevent or help treat BPH.

Even if you have BPH, with its urge to urinate more frequently, doctors advise you should drink plenty of water. Do not cut back on fluid intake. You can risk dehydration and bladder infections, and drinking lots of water keeps any retained water in the bladder diluted, decreasing the chance of dehydration and bladder infection.

Experts have also noted that caffeine, alcohol — including beer — and spicy or acidic foods can irritate the prostate, and advise patients to cut down or even eliminate these foods and drinks from their diet. Research has found that a diet heavy in soy products, sunflower seeds and pumpkin seeds may be helpful, however, as these foods seem to help eliminate the hormone

DHT that is theorized to be behind the growth of the prostate later in life. Also, B vitamins and zinc have been noted for helping prostate health in general.

Staying trim may also lessen your chances of developing BPH. One study found that men with waists larger than 43 inches are twice as likely to suffer from enlarged prostates. It's just one more reason to eat right.

Keep in mind as well that decongestants and antihistamines can exacerbate an enlarged prostate, possibly thickening its secretions as well as causing the prostate to contract, further shutting down urine flow.

And now for some really good news: Frequent whoopee-making sessions can at the least forestall prostate problems. Just thought we'd mention this before moving on to even more big trouble caused by one little gland: prostatitis.

Prostatitis can be caused by bacteria or have no known origin, but can be a vexing illness. Acute bacterial prostatitis can cause chills, lower back pain and urinary irritation. Hospitalization and intravenous treatment with antibiotics may be needed in severe cases and further treatment with drugs may be needed for a month to six weeks.

Chronic bacterial prostatitis is seen more frequently in older men. Whereas acute bacterial prostatitis is often presented by an inflamed, tender prostate, in chronic bacterial prostatitis the prostate is often normal, though "the gland can sometimes be boggy and tender," according to one source. The illness is difficult to treat because it's hard for antibiotics to be delivered into the prostate through the bloodstream. Still, successful treatment rates of 30 percent to 100 percent have been reported after three months of treatment with certain drugs.

Nonbacterial prostatitis and a condition known as prostatodynia are often confused with benign prostatic hyperplasia because many of the symptoms — weak urinary stream, the need to urinate at night, etc. — are the same. Even though bacteria have not been shown to be the causes of these conditions, there has been success treating them with antibiotics such as tetracycline and doxycycline. Though difficult to cure, "symptoms improve in up to 50 percent of treated patients," according to the American Academy of Family Physicians.

Overshadowing BPH and prostatitis, of course, is prostate cancer. This deadly cancer strikes more than 200,000 men each year and is, as previously stated, the second-leading cause of cancer death in men in the United States. Ten percent of all men are estimated to develop prostate cancer in the course of their lifetimes.

The good news is that BPH, smoking and diet are not considered huge risk factors for prostate cancer, although there is some evidence that a diet high in fats may increase the risk. A family history does pose a risk factor, as men who have a father or brother who have had the disease have a higher likelihood of developing the disease. Race is also a factor — African-Americans are more likely to develop prostate cancer and are urged to begin screening at age 40 because of this. But age is the leading risk factor for prostate cancer, as almost 70 percent of prostate cancer cases occur in men ages 65 and older.

However, outside of the risk factors noted above, screening has been a contentious process in regard to prostate cancer. The most widely used method, a test known as the prostate-specific antigen (PSA), involves looking for a marker for the disease. But the test remains controversial "because it is not yet known if this test actually saves lives," admits the National Cancer Institute (NCI).

PSA, a protein made in the prostate, is thought by some to be a biological marker for prostate cancer. The PSA test measures PSA levels in the blood and, while it's normal for men to have low levels, a higher level may be an indicator of cancer.

However, "PSA levels alone do not give doctors enough information to distinguish between benign prostate conditions and cancer," notes the NCI. "However, the doctor will take the result of the PSA test into account when deciding whether to check further for signs of prostate cancer.

"There is no specific normal or abnormal PSA level. However, the higher a man's PSA level, the more likely that cancer is present. But because various factors can cause PSA levels to fluctuate, one abnormal PSA test does not necessarily indicate a need for other diagnostic tests. When PSA levels continue to rise over time, other tests may be needed."

Contributing to the controversy is the fact that even if the PSA test does indicate the presence of a small tumor, it may be so slow-growing that it never becomes a threat to a man's life. At the same time, early detection with PSA testing may not help save the life of a man with a rapidly growing cancer that has already spread to another part of the body.

Also, false-positive test results can detect an elevated PSA level even when cancer is not present and lead to more tests such as biopsies that are expensive and can take a psychological toll on a patient and his family. "Most men with an elevated PSA test turn out not to have cancer," notes the NCI. "Only 25 percent to 30 percent of men who have a biopsy due to elevated PSA levels actually have prostate cancer." And there is also the risk of a false negative PSA test, in which a tumor can go undetected because PSA levels seem normal or unelevated.

So it's a bit of a muddle. There are no established, normal PSA levels — and yet higher levels than ordinary PSA levels make the likelihood of cancer stronger. Because of this muddle, some doctors argue against routine and regular screenings, while others suggest annual screenings for men over age 50, and at age 40 for those with risk factors.

"It is not clear if the benefits of PSA screening outweigh the risks of follow-up diagnostic tests and cancer treatments," says the NCI. "The PSA test may detect small cancers that would never become life-threatening. This situation, called overdiagnosis, puts men at risk for complications from unnecessary treatments, such as surgery or radiation."

Researchers are busy trying to solve this controversy with further analysis of the costs and benefits of PSA screening. Also, better methods of detecting and separating slow-growing cancers from fast-growing cancers are being researched, as are different ways of measuring PSA. Given the above, the best advice is talk to your doctor. Prostate cancer is nothing to take lightly, and as with all other aspects of your health, it's important to take charge and, with your doctor, determine the best course of testing.

CHAPTER 14

I Am Woman

You men can now go into the kitchen and make something healthy to eat (and stay away from the ice cream!). We're going to kvetch here for a minute about "the ladies."

We're going to talk about what they used to call "the change of life" — and all of the different issues that rise from it.

We're talking menopause.

As in "the end of menstruation as you know it," as one source puts it. "Hormone levels shift. Ovulation stops. Feelings and moods adjust. Decades of periods come to a halt. The Change of Life has arrived on the scene."

The Change of Life — they're still calling it that, apparently — usually has its onset between ages 45 and 55. Over a period of two to three years the production of the hormone estrogen, which is involved in the development of a woman's breasts and which prompts the uterus to build a lining into which a fertilized egg can nestle, begins to decrease and as it decreases the menstrual cycles become more irregular.

You might experience skipped periods, lighter or heavier menstrual flow, as well as hot flashes that cause a sensation of heat across the upper body, bright-red blushing, a change in elasticity of the skin, some thinning of the hair, problems with memory, urinary problems such as leaking or a burning sensation, mood swings, a decreased interest in sex and weight gain around your waist.

Sleeplessness and vaginal dryness in the short term may also be present while "some long-term conditions, such as osteoporosis and coronary heart disease, are more common in women in the decades after menopause," notes the National Cancer Institute.

"Many women in perimenopause (the five- to 10-year period prior to the onset of full symptoms) and menopause feel depressed and irritable," notes one expert source. "Some researchers believe that the decrease in estrogen triggers changes in your brain, causing depression. Others think that other symptoms you're having, such as sleep problems, hot flashes, night sweats and fatigue, cause these feelings. Or, it could be a combination of hormone changes and symptoms. But these symptoms could also have causes that are unrelated to menopause."

Some women enter a period of depression with menopause, suffering regret at the thought of the end of their child-bearing years, low self-esteem and negative feelings in general about the onset of menopause. On the other hand, "some women rejoice," notes one source. "They view menopause as a change all right — a change for the better! After all, they can wave a fond farewell to PMS (premenstrual syndrome), cysts, fibroids, child-rearing responsibilities and worries about pregnancy. And, the best part is FREEDOM from monthly periods."

Of course, this happy source notes of the

loss of monthly periods and the crossover to a new freedom, "It's normal to grieve for the loss of an old friend — even if she did seem to show up at the worst moments. Thirty-plus years is what you'd call a long relationship. That's why menopause can also be a time when a woman mourns the loss of her fertility and worries about aging and illness. The good news is that society and the medical community have started to view menopause as an important life event."

"Menopause causes a radical change in a woman and emotional problems are often part of the deal," notes one expert. "Whereas some may feel happy about not having to worry about unplanned pregnancies, birth control methods and monthly 'curses,' others suffer from just about every negative emotion possible. Nervousness, irritability, sudden crying jags, excessive fatigue and depression are all possible side effects of menopause."

It's important to add that in addition to the emotional trials mentioned above, postmenopausal women also are at an increased risk for bone loss — osteoporosis — and heart disease. And while the medical community is indeed starting to view menopause as an important life event, there is plenty of controversy over whether, and how, menopause and its symptoms and risks should be treated medically.

One common treatment, hormone-replacement therapy, replaces the hormones your ovaries are no longer producing and can ease the symptoms of menopause, and also help prevent bone loss and the effects of osteoporosis. However, while these prescription drugs can reduce hot flashes, reduce vaginal dryness, slow bone loss and alleviate depression and mood swings, they can also put you at greater risk of blood clots, heart attacks, stroke, breast cancer and gall bladder disease.

In fact, the National Institutes of Health decided to halt a large trial study of 16,000 healthy women, half of whom took hormones and the other half a placebo, when the combination of estrogen plus progestin increased the risk of heart disease, breast cancer, stroke and blood clots. Another study found that women aged 65 and older who took estrogen and progestin doubled their risk of developing dementia. On the other hand, incidences of hip fractures and colon cancer were reduced among the women who took the two hormones.

Studies have also found that long-term use of estrogen alone increases the risk of endometrial cancer. And a 26 percent increase in breast cancer was found among women who took estrogen in combination with progestin, with a significant increase in the spread of the cancer to other organs compared to nonusers of hormones. Likewise, women who used estrogen alone to alleviate the symptoms and effects of menopause were twice as likely to develop ovarian cancer as were women who did not take hormones, according to the NCI. The risk of ovarian cancer associated with the use of estrogen and progestin, meanwhile, was higher than for the nonusers but was "not statistically significant."

As far as heart disease, researchers found that estrogen in combination with progestin "does not protect but may increase the risk of heart disease among generally healthy postmenopausal women," reports the NCI. The study, in fact, found a 24 percent increase in heart disease among hormone users, with a whopping 81 percent increased risk in the first year of use. While there seems to be some promise in estrogen alone in protecting against heart disease, more studies are continuing to look at the hormone's effects on this disease.

Estrogen by itself and in combination with progestin has been shown to be effective in preventing the loss of bone mass and density, which can cause bones to become frail and lead to fractures. The large study done on the hormones found "a decreased risk of fracture in all subgroups of women regardless of age, smoking, fall and fracture history, past use of hormones, parental fracture history or years since menopause," the NCI said. "However, some studies have shown that the benefits on bone health disappear after short-term hormone use is discontinued. Use of estrogen for three to five years to relieve symptoms of menopause did very little to prevent fractures from osteoporosis in women when they reached ages 75 to 80. These studies suggested that women who take estrogen to maintain mineral bone density must continue taking estrogen to benefit from its effects on bone health."

There were other benefits to hormone therapy, including a 37 percent reduction in colorectal cancers. However, there was a 41 percent increase in the number of strokes among women taking estrogen and progestin, and a doubling in the incidences of blood clots.

A new method of treating the symptoms of menopause may allow your doctor to tailor your treatment. Using saliva samples gathered over the course of a month, a detailed hormonal profile can be used by doctors to create "individual hormone treatments," says one expert source.

The test is highly accurate as well as noninvasive. "It takes the guesswork out of making a proper diagnosis and allows individualized treatment with maximum benefits and minimum side effects," said Dr. Susan Lark, a top expert on women's health and nutrition.

Doctors have been reluctant to test for hormonal levels because such tests on blood, for instance, are notoriously unreliable. But the saliva test "is able to show precisely how a woman's hormone levels change throughout the month," said Dr. Lark. "Saliva is collected during the month and is then sent to be tested. The results can be used to both diagnose conditions and to help develop a specific treatment program. For instance, if a woman is having PMS symptoms, she may be not producing progesterone at all or the levels may be dropping sooner than they should. Knowing the precise levels of progesterone throughout the month means the difference between a woman taking progesterone for 12 days before her period or only seven."

Such tests, used on menopausal women, could limit the amount of hormone supplements needed and the time over which they take them, hopefully decreasing the adverse side effects detailed above.

What's the upshot of hormonal therapy for menopause?

"Women should discuss with their health care provider whether to take menopausal hormones and what alternatives may be appropriate for them," says the NCI.

What are some of these alternatives? Calcium, for one. Experts advise postmenopausal women who are not on hormone therapy to take 1,500 milligrams of calcium per day to prevent loss of bone mineral density.

A new report from the surgeon general strongly recommends staying active into adulthood to keep bones healthy and strong. The report also advises people who are at risk — such as women who have a history of osteoporosis in their families — receive a bone density test, as should all people over age 65.

Half of all Americans older than 50 will be at risk of fractures because of thinning bones by the year 2020, unless they take preventative action through diet, exercise and by getting enough calcium and vitamin D, the report said.

The report advised that people over age 50 who break a bone should be evaluated to determine if they have osteoporosis — something that is not now done, according to experts, who also note the devastating effects a broken hip, for instance, can have on an older person's life. "A hip fracture can set off a spiral leading to a nursing home and death," notes *The New York Times*. "[Twenty] percent of people who break a hip die within a year."

"One of the ideas that people have is that you earned your fracture," said Dr. Joan

McGowan, chief of the musculoskeletal branch at the National Institute of Arthritis and Musculoskeletal and Skin Diseases. "You tripped, or you were ice skating with your granddaughter ,and you fell and broke your arm. Well, how many times did your granddaughter fall and not break an arm?"

So it's important to get calcium, either through diet or through supplements. A cup of milk or calcium-fortified orange juice contains about 300 mg. Likewise, a cup of yogurt has about 400 mg., while an ounce of cheddar cheese has about 200 mg. If you can't consume the adequate amount of calcium through diet alone, calcium supplements are a great way to get it. Also, vitamin D is important in helping your body absorb calcium and the National Osteoporosis Foundation recommends getting 400 International Units per day for women — and men — ages 51 to 70 and 600 IUs for people age 70 and older. Most multivitamins contain about 400 IU of vitamin D.

Drugs for the prevention and treatment of osteoporosis are also available by prescription. Fosamax, Risedronate and Calcitonin have all been shown to be effective in slowing bone loss, increasing bone density and either reducing the risk of spine and hip fractures or easing the pain that is associated with fractures.

Another new drug, called Forteo, has been touted as a breakthrough for its ability to actually rebuild bone. A synthetic version of the parathyroid hormone, or PTH, Forteo helps increase the number of agents called osteoblasts, which help offset the loss of calcium in bone, especially in women who have low levels of estrogen.

Patients in one study of 1,637 postmenopausal women found that Forteo helped rebuild bone so successfully that most women were able to get off the drug in less than two years. The downside, however, is that users must inject the drug under their skin every day. "But patients quickly get used to that and are so pleased with the benefits that they are usually motivated to continue," said Dr. Claude Arnaud, professor emeritus of medicine and physiology at the University of California, San Francisco. And he noted that researchers are working on oral and inhaled versions of the drug.

Other therapies for the treatment of

menopausal symptoms veer into the realm of nontraditional medicine. An herbal supplement known as black cohosh has been found in some small German trial studies to reduce hot flashes — but the trials followed women for only a short period of time and the German agency that regulates black cohosh — it is not regulated by the FDA in this country — recommends not using it for longer than six months. Side effects of black cohosh can include a slowed heartbeat, visual problems, dizziness, nausea and vomiting.

Other studies, inconclusive as well, show that such touted menopausal remedies as dong quai, red clover, yam cream and chaste berry should either be avoided entirely or taken under the supervision of your doctor. Still, some nontraditional techniques to treat the symptoms of menopause — meditation, hypnosis, acupuncture and deep-breathing exercises, for instance — are showing promise, according to the National Center for Complementary and Alternative Medicine.

What else can help? Some experts advise women who are having hot flashes to avoid the triggers of a hot environment, hot or spicy foods, hot drinks, caffeine and alcohol. "Dress in layers and keep a fan in your home or workplace," advises one expert. "Regular exercise might also bring relief from hot flashes and other symptoms. Ask your doctor about taking an antidepressant medicine. There is proof that these can be helpful for some women."

Vaginal dryness can be relieved by an over-the-counter lubricant. And mood swings can be treated with exercise, by getting enough sleep and/or with the use of antidepressants. "Think about going to a support group for women who are going through the same thing as you or getting counseling to talk through your problems and fears," says an expert source.

"All women can adopt a healthy lifestyle by not smoking, exercising regularly and eating a healthy diet," notes the NCI.

Take care of yourself and be sure to let your doctor know of any health concerns.

"Menopause is a natural part of aging that is going to happen no matter what," says one expert. "In the United States alone, there are more than 30 million women who are postmenopausal. These women enjoy an active and happy life by taking care of themselves and knowing when to call for their doctor's assistance."

Women need to be very careful about two more serious obstacles to good health — breast cancer and cervical cancer.

Several risk factors "cannot be easily changed" when discussing the prevention of breast cancer, notes the American Cancer Society, including:

- *Having your first period before age 12*
- *Not having children before you are 30 years old*
- *Late onset of menopause*
- *A family history of breast cancer*

But scientists have identified some factors that can increase the risk for breast cancer:

- *The use of hormones*
- *Excessive alcohol consumption*
- *Not breastfeeding*
- *Obesity*
- *Lack of exercise*

"Some studies also suggest that diets high in vegetables and fruits decreases the risk for breast cancer, although this evidence is much weaker than for other cancer sites," the ACS says. "Alcohol increases risk to some extent, however, and exercising longer and harder may be linked to a reduced risk of breast cancer."

The best advice to prevent breast cancer, says the ACS, is to engage in "vigorous" (there's that word again) physical activity for at least four hours a week, avoid or be very moderate in your drinking (no more than a drink a day), and keep your "lifetime weight gain" to a minimum by limiting your calories and exercising.

As for testing for breast cancer, the ACS recommends the following:

● *Annual mammograms starting at age 40 and continuing as long as a woman is in good health*

● *Clinical breast exams, or CBEs, which should be part of a periodic health exam — every three years for women in their 20s and 30s and every year for women age 40 and over*

● *Women should report any breast change promptly to their doctors. Also, a breast self-exam is an option for women beginning in their 20s*

● *Women who are at increased risk, that is, there is a family history of the disease or a genetic tendency for breast cancer, should talk to their health-care providers about starting mammography screening earlier, as well as having ultrasound or MRI tests done, or having more frequent tests.*

Lastly, women need to begin cervical cancer screening at age 21 or three years after they begin having intercourse, says the ACS. Screening should be done every year with a regular Pap test or every two years with a new test, the liquid Pap test. The ACS recommends that after age 30, women who have had three normal Pap tests in a row can go to a semi-annual Pap test, every two or three years. Women ages 70 and older who have had three normal tests in a row and no abnormal tests in the previous 10 years may elect to stop screening. And women who have had a total hysterectomy — unless it was done as a treatment for cervical cancer or pre-cancer — may also elect to stop having cervical cancer screening.

Cervical cancer has largely been reduced in the United States thanks to regular Pap testing. While worldwide there are 470,000 new cases and 225,000 deaths, just 11,000 new case are expected each year in the United

States, with 4,000 deaths. And researchers are working on ways to limit that number even further, including a still-experimental vaccine that has proven 100 percent effective in preventing cervical cancer.

The vaccine works by making men and women immune to a group of common viruses transmitted by sexual intercourse, which are believed to be responsible for nearly every case of cervical cancer. Because men are carriers of the virus, experts will recommend that children of both sexes be immunized at age 9 or 10.

CHAPTER 15

The Bump
Bounce
Boogie

Eeeee-ow. Minor aches and pains are part of growing older, especially after exercise or other physical exertion. But aches and pains to your joints that just won't go away could signal something more dire: arthritis.

Swelling or stiffness in a joint upon arising in the morning, frequent pain, redness of the skin around a joint, or even unexplained fever, weight loss or weakness that lasts more than two weeks could be a signal you're suffering from arthritis.

"If left untreated or poorly managed, arthritis can be very debilitating, both physically and emotionally," notes one source. But arthritis can be successfully treated, now more than when old Uncle Bill was hobbling around on his bad knee. And by staying on top of your aches and pains and not letting a touch of arthritis worsen and get the best of you, you can maintain your quality of life — and your overall health — for years and years.

What causes arthritis? Hereditary factors are part of the cause in some people, although some people with a family history of the disease don't get it. Overuse of a joint certainly can cause it, as can pushing a joint too far and too fast following a major or even minor injury. Obesity also puts too much pressure on your joints, especially knees, and over time can lead to arthritis.

Osteoarthritis, or degenerative joint disease, affects about 21 million Americans. Most people older than age 60 show some evidence of osteoarthritis on X-rays and one-third of those will complain of pain because of it. The disease mostly affects the cartilage, which, when healthy, allows bones to glide over each other and also helps absorb shocks. If, because of injury or wear over time, the cartilage breaks down, the bones rub together causing pain, swelling and ultimately the loss of motion in a joint.

Rheumatoid arthritis, the second most common form of arthritis — it affects 2 million people in the United States — can affect other parts of the body beyond joints. It's an inflammatory disease and begins at a younger age than osteoarthritis, and also often follows a symmetrical pattern — meaning that if one knee is affected, for instance, the other will be also. Fibromyalgia, systemic lupus, erythematosus, gout and scleroderma are all forms of rheumatoid arthritis. Rheumatoid arthritis may last just a few months or a year or two, while some people may have symptoms that slowly worsen over time, leading to serious joint damage.

Can either form of arthritis be prevented?

In the case of rheumatoid arthritis, the answer is often No. With osteoarthritis, the answer is a sticky Yes.

It's sticky because every health professional in the country will tell you that one of the best things you can do to promote and maintain your health is to exercise — and yet that same exercise can be the source of your arthritis and its pain.

"Glance through almost any newspaper or magazine these days and you'll find an article extolling the benefits of sports participation," notes Dr. Edward G. McFarland, director of the Division of Adult Orthopedics at Johns Hopkins University. "Hard on the heels of these articles are others filled with dire warnings of sports-related joint injuries. If you're lucky enough to survive the injury, it seems almost certain that you'll develop osteoarthritis as a result. For those considering taking up a sport to improve their health, it's a troublesome irony.

"Exercise can cause osteoarthritis in people who develop joint injuries as a result of their sport. Such injuries can range from very common knee maladies to the relatively rare neck fracture. What these injuries have in common is that they set up inflammation in the affected joint. Inflammation can lead to damage to the cartilage, which can then lead to osteoarthritis. Such a scenario produces what's called secondary osteoarthritis, because it happens secondarily, or following an injury.

"Running and other weight-bearing exercises may place the participant particularly at risk," Dr. McFarland noted. "That's because highly repetitive, stressful exercising like running tends to wear down the protective cartilage in the joint more quickly than normal wear and tear. Some studies suggest that people,who already have some abnormalities in their joints and their alignment may be more susceptible that others to joint injuries from running."

Furthering the irony is the fact that one of the most common prescriptions for managing, as well as preventing, arthritis is ... exercise!

That's because being overweight can lead to osteoarthritis — and the best way to reduce weight is to engage in a regular exercise program. But even if you develop osteoarthritis, exercise helps tremendously in maintaining and regaining range of motion in affected joints.

One 18-month study of 252 overweight, sedentary and arthritis-inflicted people at Wake Forest University found that diet and exercise improved their physical function by 24 percent.

"Twenty years ago, physicians often advised patients with osteoarthritis to avoid exercise for fear of exacerbating symptoms," said Dr. Stephen Messier, director of the J.B. Snow Biomechanics Laboratory as well as the Wake Forest University Runner's Clinic. "We now know that this was not the best advice. Today's standard of care for physicians is to advise patients to exercise. Why put more stress on a knee that already hurts? We found in (the) study that the diet and exercise group actually decreased their pain by 30 percent, even though they put more stress on their joints.

"How can that happen? There are a number of possible explanations. One, muscles get stronger and are therefore better able to absorb the shock normally absorbed by the bones. Two, the mechanics are better, so they are not putting stress where it shouldn't be. Three, we found that inflammation decreases. We think now that inflammatory biomarkers called cytokines, which degrade cartilage, decrease in number."

However, continuing to pound a joint after a sports injury to a knee, for instance, is probably not a good idea, noted Dr. McFarland. He suggests switching to an exercise you're more comfortable with, such as a switch from a high-impact sport like running to a relatively lower-impact sport like bicycling, to preserve cartilage and protect the joint from further injury.

But he supported the findings of the Wake Forest University study. "It is most certainly true that people who find an exercise that works for them will preserve joint functioning better over time than those who cease to exercise," he said. "Regular exercise will keep your muscles in good shape and help stabilize affected joints, and you'll feel better, both physically and mentally. So if you've had a diagnosis of osteoarthritis, find an exercise you enjoy and are comfortable doing. In the long run it will benefit you greatly."

Another expert source notes the importance of three kinds of exercises for treating arthritis:

● **Range-of-motion exercises.** These have

you move your joint as far as possible in all directions, helping you avoid stiffness and keeping your joints flexible.

● **Strengthening exercises.** Lifting and resistance exercises strengthen joints and the muscles surrounding them.

● **Endurance exercises.** Walking, water exercises and stationary bicycles all help build up your endurance in a low-impact fashion to minimize further cartilage loss.

"Walking strengthens muscles in the lower body, helps to build new joint and bone tissue and helps to ward off or slow osteoporosis," notes the U.S. Administration on Aging (USAA). "Other aerobic exercises as well as exercises that increase flexibility should be included in your routine. Other good aerobic exercises for weight-bearing joints include dancing, tennis, racquetball, basketball and biking."

If you have arthritis, swimming, in particular, is excellent for its treatment. "It offers many of the benefits of other aerobic exercises without putting undue stress on joints which, because of arthritis or injury, are unable to repair and build themselves in the normal manner," notes the USAA.

If you are overweight, losing weight is one of the best things you can do to ease your arthritis symptoms and to help your overall health. "Studies have shown that overweight women who lost an average of 11 pounds substantially reduced the development of osteoarthritis," noted one source. As mentioned above, excessive weight puts strain on joints as well as other organs in your body, such as your heart. Shedding weight can also make it easier for you to get into and stay in shape.

Conventional medicine has also come up with various pain relievers. NSAIDS, non-inflammatory and nonsteroidal drugs, are available by prescription or as over-the-counter remedies, while COX-2 inhibitors can cause fewer problems in the digestive tract than NSAIDS and can be a good alternative to them. Non-narcotic relievers such as aspirin and acetaminophen are generally available without a prescription. And there are some topical creams that can be applied directly on a painful joint to provide relief.

Arthritis pain in the knee from osteoarthritis is also being treated with something called hyaluronan (HA) supplementation therapy.

In the procedure, hyaluronic acid, a naturally occurring substance found in joint fluid, is injected into the affected knee — and while 40 percent of patients say it gives good pain relief, an amazing 25 percent report a 100 percent improvement and become completely pain-free.

"We know it decreases pain by working on nerve endings to reduce inflammation," said Dr. Roy Altman, a professor of rheumatology at UCLA Medical School and the author of a new study on the procedure. "When you inject hyaluronan into a knee, it acts like a sponge and absorbs the enzymes that break down cartilage."

Dr. Altman said tests in France and England also reveal that hyaluronan show promise in promoting the growth of new cartilage. The procedure is also benefiting people who can't take NSAIDS because of their effect on the digestive tract — and studies are showing promise as well for other parts of the body that are prone to arthritis, such as shoulders, elbows, ankles and hips. "This is a welcome addition to the treatment of osteoarthritis," said Dr. Altman. "The results are very promising."

As for the pain from rheumatoid arthritis, many pain-relieving drugs have been tried with varying success. But one new drug, Humira, is letting patients take control of their own therapy. Unlike other drugs for rheumatoid arthritis, such as Enbrel — which is administered by a doctor twice a week — and Remicade — which requires an IV infusion every eight weeks in a hospital — Humira is administered once a week by the patient, at home.

Researchers have found that people with rheumatoid arthritis have an excess of a certain protein that can trigger inflammation as part of the body's normal immune system response. The immune system mistakenly attacks healthy tissue, especially in the tissues that lines and cushions joints, leading to inflammation and, over time, joint damage. Humira blocks the offending protein and in some cases improvement is shown within a day as inflammation subsides and the pain eases.

In less chronic cases of osteoarthritis, some old remedies still stand up to scrutiny. Heat and cold can also be used to treat the pain from arthritis. An ice pack wrapped in a towel and applied to the affected area can help reduce swelling and relieve pain. Heat treatments such as a warm bath or shower, or a heating pad placed on the joint for about 15 minutes, can help relieve pain.

Massage, in the hands of a trained therapist, can also improve circulation to an affected area, reduce inflammation and relieve pain. But make sure the therapist is familiar with your type and location of arthritis.

Can vitamins help arthritis? Some experts say yes, pointing in particular to vitamin C, which helps in the formation of collagen, a component of cartilage. "A further benefit of vitamin C is that it is a powerful antioxidant that helps mop up damaging free radicals, which are produced during the inflammatory processes," notes an article in *Healthy Way* magazine. Another source says vitamin C also helps heal wounds and repair connective tissues.

Research, according to *Healthy Way*, also suggests that osteoarthritis progresses more slowly in people who have a high intake of vitamin D — which, we will remember from the discussions of osteoporosis, helps the body absorb calcium. Vitamin E, meanwhile, is cited by some as another good method to help repair sports injuries, as it sops up the free radicals produced by damaged muscles.

Can the supplements glucosamine or chondroitin, pushed by many health-food stores as an alternative method of building cartilage, actually help? Perhaps. "One study from Europe actually showed that after three years, joint space was improved, suggesting cartilage buildup," noted Dr. Stephen Messier of Wake Forest University. "Our hypothesis is that glucosamine and chondroitin will relieve pain and improve function in the joint by building cartilage and making the cartilage more pliable. People who exercise and take the supplement are going to get added benefit." But he added that since the supplements are still so new, there's little knowledge about any long-term adverse effects of these supplements.

Other sources indicate that a diet rich in the omega-3 fatty acids — salmon and mackerel are good sources, and it also comes in capsules — can relieve sore joints and morning stiffness; manganese ascorbate can help build connective tissue such as cartilage; aloe vera is touted for having natural anti-inflammatory agents, and the herb Urtica dioica helps your body get rid of uric acid and other acid metabolites that can cause pain by collecting around a joint.

Flaxseed, which comes in capsules, meal, flour, seeds or as an oil, may relieve pain and inflammation, according to *The Arthritis Foundation's Guide to Alternative Therapies*. And 1,800 mg per day of GLA oil capsules may also ease pain, inflammation and stiffness.

"There is a handful of supplements which have been shown in clinical research trials to help with the pain and inflammation of arthritis, but many others have not," said Judith Horstman, author of the Arthritis Foundation guide.

Horstman singled out Arnica, Aconite, Adrenal extracts, spleen extracts, thymus extracts, Autumn crocus, GHB, Chaparral and Kombucha tea as supplements that should especially be used with caution. And of course, you should check with your doctor before taking any kind of supplement.

CHAPTER 16

Beneath Still Waters

If the eyes are the window into the soul, our skin is a billboard advertising all sorts of information about us and our overall health. Wrinkles, spots and dry skin can all signal to ourselves and others that we're younger than we look — and perhaps not as healthy as we ought to be or want to be.

And skin is something that's easy to maintain — and just as easy to wreck.

"Americans spend billions of dollars each year on skin-care products that promise to ease wrinkles, lighten age spots and eliminate itching, flaking or redness," notes the National Institute on Aging. "But the simplest and cheapest way to keep your skin healthy and young-looking is to stay out of the sun."

Stay out of the sun. Any cosmetic surgeon or dermatologist will tell you just how great the sun and its damaging effects have been for their business, yet every summer our beaches are a sea of reddening, tanning, increasingly at-risk bodies. But ironically, even as we catch rays and chase after that perfect tan to enhance our looks, the sun is doing irreparable damage to our skin that will eventually prematurely age us — and perhaps even prematurely kill us.

"Sunlight is a major cause of the skin changes we think of as aging — changes such as wrinkles, dryness and age spots," says one expert source. "Your skin does change with age. For example, you sweat less, leading to increased dryness. As your skin ages, it becomes thinner and loses fat, so it looks less plump and smooth. Underlying structures — veins and bones in particular — become more prominent. Your skin can take longer to heal when injured.

"You can delay these changes by staying out of the sun. Although nothing can completely undo sun damage, the skin can sometimes repair itself. So, it's never too late to protect yourself from the harmful effects of the sun."

Dr. Robert Kotler, a prominent Beverly Hills cosmetic surgeon and the author of *Confessions of a Beverly Hills Cosmetic Surgeon*, advises people to stop smoking and to stay out of the sun as well.

"A wrinkle is like a crack or a fault in the skin," he said. "Consider the skin as a kind of a cloth-like material. What happens is it kind of tears right below the surface, due to sun and due to cigarette smoking and unhealthy lifestyles.

"The collagen fibers, which are kind of like the core constituent in the skin, break down. It's like a rubber band that gets stretched out. And there is literally a lethal effect from ultraviolet light. And that's why sunscreens work. It prevents the sun from breaking down the constituents, the building blocks of the skin.

"Protect your skin from excess sun. That doesn't mean you can't go out without a hat for 15 or 20 minutes. But after 20 minutes, light-skinned people will notice their skin starts to get a little red. And that's the first sign of skin damage.

"The second sign of skin damage is a tan. People don't realize that every time you tan, that is proof that you've damaged your skin. What happens is that nature mobilizes, knowing that you're sitting in the sun too much. The body mobilizes whatever pigment you have to come out and protect you.

"But what happens is hat that 15- or 20-year-old kid who loves to be tan, 20 years down the line starts to look like a prune, because each one of those tanning episodes gives a little bit of death to the skin."

Heredity also plays a part in how much damage the sun can do to your skin, Dr. Kotler said. "How much pigment you have in your skin also determines how much you're going to wrinkle," he added. "The closer your ancestors were to the equator — for instance, the Middle East or Northern Africa — the more people have darker skin and don't wrinkle as much. On the other hand, if you're from Finland or Norway, with fair, white skin and blue eyes, you're a sitting duck for skin deterioration. The skin is so fair, it has very little of the pigment melanin. That's nature's great protection."

Beyond the purely cosmetic changes that can occur from sun damage and aging itself, what should you be aware of regarding your skin?

Well, first, of course, is skin cancer.

It's one of the most common cancers in the United States, with 40 percent to 50 percent of Americans having it at least once in their lifetimes. Ultraviolet radiation from the sun is the greatest factor in the development of skin cancer and take note that even the artificial sources of ultraviolet radiation, that from tanning booths and sun lamps, can also cause skin cancer. As seems obvious, people who live in the Sunbelt — the South and Southwest — are more prone to skin cancer, as opposed to those in the sun-challenged Upper Midwest and Northwestern United States.

Basal cell carcinoma is the most common skin cancer, accounting for nine in 10 cases of skin cancer in the United States. The good news about this type of skin cancer is that it is slow-growing and rarely spreads to other parts of the body. Squamous cell carcinoma also rarely spread, but are slightly more dangerous than basal cell.

The most virulent of all skin cancers is melanoma, which can and often does spread to other organs in the body and often with fatal results.

Experts recommend that you check your skin regularly and take note of any changes, such as a new growth or mole or a sore that doesn't heal. Seldom painful, skin cancers can begin as a small, smooth or shiny lump or as a firm red lump that can bleed or develop a crust on it. It can also begin growth as a small red patch that is rough, dry or scaly. If you note the appearance of any such growths on your skin, check with a doctor if the growth doesn't go away within two weeks.

The basic treatment for any skin cancer is to destroy and/or remove it from the body. This often means cutting the growth away from your body and in some cases the treatment can include radiation or even chemotherapy. The type of cancer, a person's age, the location of the cancer — they all come into play when considering the best treatment option.

In summation, skin cancer is nothing to fool around with. Be sensible about risks, as with any obvious and common health threat. The best prevention is to stay out of the sun, especially when its rays are the strongest at midday, or at least to wear a hat and use a proven sunblock that will block all ultraviolet radiation. And remember that while the sun's rays bring life to this earth, they can also bring death.

Exposure to the sun can do other, less life-threatening damage to your skin. Age spots — "liver spots" to some — are also caused by the sun. Known in medical terms as solar lentigo, they appear in fair-skinned people, often on the greatest areas of exposure to the sun — hands, face, arms, back and feet. There are some skin creams, "fade" creams, that can be used to eliminate these disfiguring spots and doctors also use freezing or laser treatments to remove them.

Wrinkling, meanwhile, may not be life-threatening — but it is an indication that your skin, the body's largest organ, is not healthy.

"Skin distortion is often the most visible sign of human aging," notes one publication. "The passage of time can wreak havoc on the face; leaving wrinkles, age spots and sagging skin in its wake."

"We have all seen people whose skin looks younger than their chronological age and others whose skin appears older than their years," notes *Life Extension* magazine. "You can take the initiative and minimize the impact of the environmental factors under your control. You can also utilize effective therapies to counteract changes in the skin that occur over time."

After sun exposure, cigarette smoking is the largest cause of wrinkling, says Dr. Kotler. "Cigarette smoke, with its nicotine and carbon dioxide (among other noxious elements), causes the skin's blood vessels to constrict and narrow, and thus chokes off the flow of oxygen and other nutrients to the skin," notes Dr. Kotler.

"That means less blood flow to the largest organ in the body, the skin. That's why smokers' skin looks older, more wrinkled and is of poorer quality. With every cigarette, the skin dies a little.

"The blood vessels bring the nutrients to the skin and, when you smoke, these same vessels bring noxious elements like carbon monoxide and carbon dioxide to the skin. They're killers. Plus, the blood vessels can be shrunk by the elements in cigarette smoke, further depriving the skin of nutrients."

Besides not smoking and limiting exposure to direct sunlight, moisturizers are a great way to prevent or allay wrinkles, Dr. Kotler says. And of course, eating right and getting enough rest also help protect the skin from breaking down and wrinkling.

Experts say what you eat can be an important factor in your skin's health. "It's definitely true that diet can play an important role in all skin conditions — not just helping combat wrinkles and lines, but other skin problems as well, including acne, eczema, psoriasis — even dry flaking or very oily skin," says biochemist Dr. Elaine Linker.

Dr. Nicholas V. Perricone, author of *The Wrinkle Cure*, says omega-3 fatty acids — those found in fish oils and nuts — are vital to healthy skin, because they help reduce the body's production of inflammatory compounds.

And experts recommend avoiding foods that can sharply raise insulin levels, including the simple white sugars found in white bread and starchy foods. "Any food that causes insulin to spike can induce inflammation — and that can irritate any skin condition influenced by inflammation, which is pretty much all skin conditions, including the way skin ages," says Dr. Linker.

Foods rich in vitamin A — such as cantaloupe or sweet potatoes — can work almost as well as common, vitamin-enriched topical treatments, some experts say.

"Eating foods rich in vitamin A or beta-carotene is not going to give as powerful (a) cell turnover effect as a prescription vitamin A cream, but these foods do help regulate cell turnover — essentially by giving skin what it needs to perform as best as it possibly can," says Dr. Ann Yelmokas McDermott, a nutritionist at the Jean Mayer USDA Human Nutrition Center on Aging at Tufts University.

Other vitamins are essential to healthy

skin as well, says Dr. Perricone. Antioxidants such as vitamin B complex, C and E can create a "safety net" for your skin by helping reduce the environmental factors that can damage your skin's membrane.

"Taking just one nutrient alone will not give you good skin," says Dr. Linker. "You have to have a balance, which is essential not only to the health of your skin, but it prevents an imbalance from occurring — and an imbalance is what contributes to inflammation."

Experts advise a varied diet rich in the following can help you overcome a skin problem and prevent others from occurring:

Seafood. Some experts advise eating salmon, tuna or mackerel three times a week. They recommend you eat a variety of fish as a good source of omega-3 fatty acids. "Studies show adding fish to your diet can also help reduce the inflammation associated with psoriasis and even eczema," notes one source.

Nuts, seeds and grains. One ounce of walnuts can give you the same amount of omega-3s as 3.5 ounces of salmon steak. Flax seed also is a good source of omega-3 fatty acids.

Olive oil. Use at least two tablespoons a day as a salad dressing, or use olive oil in place of other oils in cooking.

Fruit. Tomatoes, watermelon, blueberries and strawberries are all good sources of the antioxidant lycopene, which is important in maintaining healthy skin.

Vegetables. Eat a wide variety of vegetables to get the full benefit of their antioxidants.

Whole-grain cereals and breads. The key is to replace white flour with whole grains to reduce the inflammatory reaction that can harm skin.

Brazil nuts, turkey and tuna. These selenium-rich foods can help reduce the inflammations in acne.

Tea. Teas — green or black — have anti-inflammatory properties that can be beneficial to skin.

Also, experts advise that you should drink plenty of **water** — between one and two quarts per day, according to Dr. Linker.

Dr. Kotler also says moisturizers can have great benefits in keeping skin healthy.

"Moisturizing helps," he said. "The skin does best when it's not dried out. Moisturizers are excellent." Dr. Kotler recommends Retin-A and says if it's used daily starting in one's 30s, it can help reduce the formation of wrinkles. Studies of Retin-A and other prescription-strength vitamin A derivatives have shown that these products can fade age spots, make wrinkles less noticeable and perhaps even prevent some precancerous changes in your skin.

But debate still rages as to whether vitamin-enhanced moisturizers help get rid of wrinkles. Some sources claim they can, while others claim they're just a marketing gimmick. "The positive effects resulting (from) the topical application of vitamin C were singled out in a recent investigation where it was proven to stimulate collagen production," one article recently claimed.

Another study was said to have "confirmed vitamin C's efficacy in improving the overall look and feel of the skin. Clinical evaluation of wrinkling, pigmentation, inflammation and hydration was performed prior to the study and at weeks 4, 8, and 12 on individuals who applied topical vitamin C complex on one-half of the face and placebo gel to the opposite side. The results showed a statistically significant improvement to the skin on the vitamin C side, with biopsies showing increased collagen formation and reduced wrinkling."

Vitamins E and A in topical form have also been studied, with some effect on skin roughness and wrinkle depth noted. But claims about the usefulness of moisturizers with vitamin additives are still being greeted with skepticism by many experts.

"Unfortunately, the sizes of the molecules of the main ingredients within nearly all moisturizers are far too large to allow them to penetrate through the skin barrier to where they are most needed," says an article in *Total Health*. "Moisturizers are not absorbed into the skin nor can they do a lot of other things that have been claimed for them, such as shrinking pores, preventing wrinkles or rejuvenating skin. In general, they serve to promote smoothness and softness by locking in whatever moisture is naturally present in the skin and retarding further loss."

Some experts point to plain petroleum jelly as a good moisturizer. Otherwise, "regular use of any supermarket or pharmacy house brand moisturizer will suffice," the article noted. "Expensive so-called finest department store brands provide little more than fancier packaging."

There are, however, some topical agents that are "worth trying," according to Dr. Nelson Lee Novick, an associate clinical professor of dermatology at The Mount Sinai School of Medicine in New York City.

Novick said that products containing alpha hydroxy acids (AHAs) might work as part of a rejuvenating program for your skin, as these AHAs are believed to work below the surface of the skin to repair damage from sun or other causes. AHAs might also stimulate the formation of new collagen, he reports. "After six months to a year of continuous application, you should see diminished sagging and less wrinkling," he wrote in *Total Health*.

That's the skinny on skin and what you can — and should — do to keep it healthy and even turn back the clock a little on the damage that's been done.

CHAPTER 17

Feed Your Head

When ditzy old Aunt Sadie became even more forgetful, when Uncle Bob started having trouble remembering people's names, we'd chalk it up to "old age" or "senior moments," just another part of the inevitable decline people experience as they grow older.

But new research is showing that not

only are such declines not inevitable — they can also be prevented in some cases and at least forestalled in others.

Though researchers have found that the brain decreases in weight and volume over time — perhaps as much as 20 percent between ages 45 and 85 as the brain loses neurons and cell fluid — a surprising number of people "function normally even when they age," says one source. "The causes of loss of memory, concentration, focus and the inability to function independently as man ages may not only be due to the aging itself as previously thought. It may be due to a combination of other brain-unhealthy behavior and habits, insufficient mental stimulation, limited thought- or response-control strategies, inadequate supplements, (or) lack of novel experiences, lack of sufficient social interactions and cooperation."

As researchers examine the ways in which the brain ages and whether social interaction, diet and other factors can be manipulated to prevent or delay such aging, such common disorders as depression are also being looked at in new light, as chemical and biological changes and other factors come into play and new treatments become available. The role of the brain, long overlooked as a player in physical health, has never been so prominent in medical research and theory as it is now.

Scientists are also noting now how exercise benefits the mind, how certain vitamins seem to be effective in alleviating some psychological or brain disorders and even noting how working hard to maintain a positive mental outlook on life can help a person's overall health — and even longevity.

Here, we're going to look at some of the psychological and brain disorders that could affect you as you pass age 40 — and some of the things you can do to try to prevent, treat or simply live with the conditions.

DEPRESSION

Though not just a disorder that strikes the middle-age or elderly, depression can often be linked to life events and traumas that can trigger it, even in middle age. The loss of a job, of a spouse, a chronic illness, divorce, a "midlife crisis" — these and other factors, including heredity, personality traits and drug and alcohol abuse — can contribute to the development of depression from middle age on.

"People used to think it was 'all in your head' and that if you really tried, you could 'pull yourself out of it,' " notes the esteemed Mayo Clinic. "Doctors now know that depression is not a weakness and you can't treat it on your own. It's a medical disorder with a biological or chemical basis."

Indeed, researchers are finding that chemical imbalances in the brain may play a large role in triggering depression. Experts have also found that in 15 percent of depression cases, the condition is a response to an illness such as cancer or Parkinson's disease, heart disease or stroke — and long-term use of some medications, including those for blood pressure and arthritis, can cause depression. An underactive thyroid gland and vitamin deficiencies have also been linked to depression — making the old-school, pull-yourself-up-by-the-bootstraps attitude toward the disease that much more absurd.

Depression is more common in women by a ratio of 2 to 1 — but 3 million to 4 million men are affected by depression. It's an equal opportunity disorder, cutting across boundaries of class, race and education.

Depression can also come out of nowhere, leaving you aware of a malaise or black cloud hovering over your days but unaware that you have a serious disorder that can, and should, be treated.

Experts have identified two main markers of depression. One is a loss of interest and pleasure in day-to-day activities. The other is simply a "depressed mood" — feelings of sadness, helplessness or despair that may be so bad they leave you in tears.

Other troubles go hand-in-hand with depression. Sleep disturbances, a large weight gain or loss, impaired concentration, a feeling of fatigue, low self-esteem, a decreased appetite for sex, thoughts of suicide or reckless behavior such as driving erratically or threats of violence to others are often also present and can help your doctor diagnose your depression.

Depression also manifests itself physically, beyond feelings of fatigue, and can lead to itching, blurred vision, stomach problems, headache or backache.

"Unlike normal sadness or grieving, most bouts of depression last for weeks, months or even years," notes Johns Hopkins University *Health After 50* library.

"Although depression is usually not considered life-threatening, it can lead to thoughts of and attempts at suicide. As many as 70 percent of suicides in the United States are related to depression and nearly 9 percent of severely depressed people commit suicide."

Generally, diagnosis of depression is based on physical and psychological evaluations and the appearances of most or all of the above markers of depression for more than two weeks. Psychotherapy "is as effective as drugs in mild cases," according to Johns Hopkins. Psychotherapy may also be used in conjunction with drugs.

Drug therapy may include the use of selective serotonin reuptake inhibitors, serotonin and norepinephrine reuptake inhibitors, all of which can rebalance the chemicals in your brain that may be causing your depression. Antidepressants, or stimulants such as Ritalin, may help.

"Medications can relieve symptoms of depression and have become the first line of treatment for most types of the disorder," notes one expert. "A combination of medications and a brief course of psychotherapy usually is effective if you have mild to moderate depression."

Doctors first work to ease the symptoms of depression, but full treatment with drugs and psychotherapy can last six months to a year to prevent a relapse. "Episodes of depression recur in the majority of people who have one episode, but continuing treatment for at least six months greatly reduces your risk of a rapid relapse."

Keep in mind that it often takes two to eight weeks for drug therapy to take hold. If the drug treatment chosen by your doctor based upon your symptoms doesn't work by the end of two months, another drug may be tried. But experts urge patients to continue taking their medications, even if you feel better, and also to make sure you see your doctor regularly so your progress can be monitored.

Also, it's important to note that there are things you should be doing during an episode of depression that can help you overcome the disorder. Avoid alcohol or other drugs, stay involved in normal day-to-day activities so you don't become isolated and, perhaps most importantly, take care of yourself. Get plenty of rest, eat right and exercise, which has been found to be an effective tool in easing stress and helping people relax.

Can depression be prevented? If the underlying cause is a genetic predisposition or chemical imbalance, probably not, and at some point in life, depression might rear its ugly head. What's important in these instances is to recognize and appreciate that you are not to blame for your depression, that there are underlying causes that are beyond your control. The sooner you recognize depression in yourself and seek treatment for it, the sooner you'll be able to get on with your life.

There are things people can do to help themselves, however, whether they're biologically or chemically predisposed to depression or not. One of the most important, research has found, is to stay connected to the world as much as possible.

We are social animals, but sometimes events occur that can strip us of our social settings. This can include the loss of a job, a divorce or the death of a spouse. It's normal to take time to oneself after such traumatic events in an effort to understand what has happened and how life will now be different. But ultimately, science has found that people who can stay connected to the world, find new avenues to new friends, new jobs, even new spouses, are mentally healthier than those who shut themselves off.

One study, done at the Harvard School of Public Health, involved a poll of 2,761 residents of New Haven, Connecticut, ages 65 and older. Seniors who took part in group pleasures with others live an average of two-and-a-half years longer than those who don't, the study found.

The most outgoing of the seniors were 19 percent less likely to die over the 13-year period studied than were those who remained isolated. Lisa Berkman, chair of the department of health and social behavior at Harvard, said the findings of the study boost two theories regarding longevity and sociability.

The first is that social activity helps the immune system. "There's a lot of physical evidence for this," Berkman said. The second theory is that social contact activates the brain, resulting in the release of natural opiates that have a calming effect and which create a sense of well-being.

Berkman says it doesn't matter what you do to stay connected — just as long as you do something.

"There is no one social activity that is key to a long life," she says, "but rather maintain ties across the board. Whether it's relatives, close friends or religious organizations, these ties have a beneficial effect on the quality and length of life.

"If you're single, having close friends is good. If you belong to a lot of volunteer organizations, that can substitute for religious organizations. What's important is that the behavior has meaning to the person who does it. Just sending a check doesn't count."

Volunteering, in fact, has benefits beyond just getting out and helping in a group setting. One study found the very act of giving — the "helper's high" in the words of Arizona State University psychologist Robert Cialdini — can help a person live longer.

One study at the University of Michigan followed 423 couples for five years. Those who said they'd helped others during the life of the study were half as likely to have died as those who didn't aid others. Even after accounting for factors such as wealth, age, smoking, drinking and exercise habits, there was a strong tie between giving and living longer.

Another Harvard study had similar results. The study, performed by the Harvard Center for Society and Health, studied 28,369 male health professionals and investigated the effects of social ties, death and heart disease. Men who had a large number of friends, relatives and other social ties lived longer than isolated peers, the study reported.

During the course of the 10-year study, 1,365 of the men died from heart disease, cancer or another cause. Men who were more socially isolated were nearly 20 percent more likely to die from any cause than their socially active peers, the study reported.

Socially isolated men were also 53 percent more likely to die from a heart-related cause. The more isolated men were also twice as likely to die from suicide or from accident than the social men, the study said.

And the isolated men had an 82 percent greater risk of death from heart disease — heart-stopping numbers in anyone's book!

For those who poke fun at marriage, there was this sobering statistic: Married men were more than two times less likely to die from suicide or accident than their single comrades.

"Staying healthy and living longer is not simply a matter of practicing good health habits or getting good medical care," said Dr. Ichiro Kawachi, director of the center and the author of the study. "A good friend can keep the doctor away."

Dr. Kawachi said it makes sense that the results would be similar among women as well and urged health-care workers to "pay attention to their clients' social situation as much as their cholesterol levels or blood pressure levels."

And a little more about those married men — a British study found that married men and women, especially those on their first or only marriage, live longer than their bachelor and bachelorette counterparts.

Researchers at Warwick University followed thousands of British men and women over a 10-year period. They found that the people who were married at the study's beginning or those who married for the first time during the course of the study were more likely to be alive at the end of the 10 years than those who never married.

"Marriage has benefits," says economics professor Andrew Oswald, who co-directed the study. "Marrying adds three years on average to you life, and you are likely to have much better health."

ALZHEIMER'S DISEASE

Strong social relationships may also be a factor in at least forestalling the debilitating effects of Alzheimer's disease. However, there are still many things that are unknown about this disease.

What are the first symptoms of Alzheimer's disease (AD)? Simple forgetfulness — a name, a place, where they put the car keys — and perhaps some trouble doing simple math problems. There may also be problems remembering simple words, some disorientation as to time and place, decreased judgment or trouble with something as easy as balancing a checkbook.

Also, a person in the first stages of AD "may put things in unusual places: an iron in the freezer or a wristwatch in the sugar bowl," notes the Alzheimer's Association. Increasingly, changes in mood — "from calm to tears to anger" — is being seen as a hallmark of Alzheimer's, as can a change in personality that makes them suspicious, confused or fearful. And a classic hallmark of AD is a loss of initiative. "The person with Alzheimer's disease may become very passive, sitting in front of the television for hours, sleeping more than usual or not wanting to do usual activities," says the association.

Can Alzheimer's be prevented? Science won't know until AD's causes can be discovered.

"Scientists do not yet fully understand what causes AD," says a report from the Alzheimer's Disease Education & Referral Center (ADEAR). "There probably is not one single cause, but several factors that affect each person differently."

Obviously, age is a huge risk factor, although one rare form of the disease, familial AD, can strike some people between ages 30 and 60. Otherwise, the number of people with the most common form, late-onset AD, doubles for every five years beyond age 65.

Scientists believe that genetics might play a role in many cases of AD, but to date have discovered just one gene that can be identified as a risk factor for the disease. For that reason, diet, education, environment and other factors are being studied to determine what, if any role, they may have in the development of the disease.

That said, there is "increasing evidence that some of the risk factors for heart disease and stroke, such as high blood pressure, high cholesterol and low levels of the vitamin folate, may predispose people to AD," says ADEAR. "Evidence for physical, mental and social activities as protective factors against AD is also increasing."

Some researchers, in fact, are finding that memory loss, Alzheimer's and other signs of a decline in brain function may be forestalled or even eliminated in those without a genetic predisposition toward the disease.

"After 40," notes one medical source, "taking up a new language or any new course of art classes, whether joining a formal class or learning on your own, is beneficial. As long as you learn something new, the nerve cells in your brain will grow and the connection between them will continue to strengthen."

Taking up woodworking, art classes and similar activities "help strengthen the part of the brain that controls spatial relations, the ability to recognize how things piece together," says the source.

Likewise, you can sharpen your hand-eye coordination and reflexes with such games as table tennis, badminton and the like — or by taking up or continuing to play a musical instrument. Reading books and a good variety of magazines and newspapers, and working hard to remember what is said in them, keeps your brain active. Games such as chess, cards and Scrabble are also good for retention of brain power, as are crossword, jigsaw and other puzzles.

You may also be able to take steps to preserve brain function by using the right combination of exercise, vitamins and foods, says Dr. Jeff Victoroff, author of *Saving Your Brain, A Revolutionary Plan to Boost Brain Power, Improve Memory* and *Protect Yourself Against Aging and Alzheimer's.*

Dr. Victoroff said the following activities, foods and supplements may help people forestall or ward off a decline in brain function.

● **Aerobic exercise.** "We've known for years that folks who are physically fit protect themselves from heart disease, but in addition, we've recently found that people who have less heart disease also have less Alzheimer's disease," said Dr. Victoroff. "If you can protect your body as a whole from vascular disease, you can also protect it from Alzheimer's." Plus, he said, "There is some research that indicates that aerobic exercise actually incorporates new neurons into the brain."

A brisk 30-minute walk each day will be enough, but other forms of exercise, even dancing, work as well.

● **Take your vitamins.**

● **Learn a new skill.** "Take a class in something you've never studied before," Dr. Victoroff said. "These are skills you've not developed and your brain will turn on and rev up in the course of new learning."

● **Drink white wine.** Although any type of alcohol, including beer, will boost your brain power, Dr. Victoroff suggests white wine because it has the fewest side effects.

"It seems that the people who have a drink or two of liquor or a glass or two of wine several times a week have a higher level of cognitive function than those who don't," he said.

● **Eat fish.** Eating fatty fish four times a week will lower your risk of developing Alzheimer's.

● **Avoid obesity.** "Keeping your weight down is important because you need to avoid adult onset diabetes, vascular disease and hypertension. All come with obesity and all are connected with brain power," said Dr. Victoroff.

● **Get plenty of sleep.** "Obviously all of us need rest, but the people who are at greatest risk for losing brain cells are those who have sleep apnea and don't know it," said Dr. Victoroff. They are usually middle-age males who snore excessively and drive their wives crazy. They need to see a doctor and get a proper diagnosis, because if they have sleep apnea, they could be killing their brain cells.

● **Keep your blood pressure in the normal range.** "Avoiding high blood pressure is immensely important," Dr. Victoroff said.

"It's not important just because it helps the vascular part of the brain, but there is very strong evidence that high blood pressure increases your risk of Alzheimer's disease."

Indeed, researchers have found a link between high cholesterol and high blood pressure and Alzheimer's disease. A Finnish study done between 1972 and 1987 found that people with high blood pressure in midlife were 2.3 times more likely to develop Alzheimer's disease, and that those with high blood pressure and high cholesterol were 3.5 times more likely to develop the disease.

Researchers are also beginning to use powerful cholesterol-lowering drugs to stop the development of Alzheimer's disease. A study at three hospitals analyzed the records of 57,000 patients and found that the patients taking statins, such as Mevacor or Pravschol, were up to 73 percent less likely to develop Alzheimer's disease.

Dr. Benjamin Wolozin, associate professor of pharmacology at Loyola University Medical Center, said the statins seem to combat Alzheimer's disease simply by improving the circulation of blood —

"including that to the brain." Dr. Wolozin urged anyone with elevated cholesterol levels to talk to their doctors about using statins, as opposed to other less-powerful anti-cholesterol agents.

"In unpublished data from our study, we found that all types of statins reduced the risk of mental impairment, but other types of (cholesterol-lowering drugs) did not," Dr. Wolozin said. This data not only shows promise in the prevention of Alzheimer's disease — it also highlights one more benefit that a low-fat diet and plenty of exercise can have on your overall health.

New drugs are also being developed to minimize the effects of Alzheimer's disease on the brain. One, Exelon, has shown benefits in memory, overall functioning and in behavior in patients with early Alzheimer's. It also helped patients who did not respond to other treatments. "People need to know that treatment in the early stages of the illness offers the best chance of successfully delaying Alzheimer's disease symptoms," said Dr. Steven Potkin, a professor at the University of California, Irvine.

Exelon is a member of a class of drugs

known as Cholinesterase inhibitors, which also includes the drugs Aricept and Reminyl. The drugs are believed to slow mental deterioration by boosting the function of a brain chemical called acetylcholine.

"We see either improvement or stabilization in functional abilities, whether it's using the telephone, making change or being able to get from one place to another," said Dr. Rachelle Doody, an associate professor in the department of neurology at Baylor College of Medicine.

The drugs are effective for six months to two years and, while memory can improve, the best effect the drugs have is slowing the onset of Alzheimer's disease, experts note. For that reason, as in all other aspects of your health, it's important to stay on top of any symptoms you experience or you see a spouse experiencing so effective treatment can begin as soon as possible.

"The earlier the diagnosis, the earlier treatment can be started and the more the patient can benefit," said Dr. John Morris, a national board member of the Alzheimer's Association. "Don't wait until the patient is at an advanced stage ready for the nursing home because of the mistaken belief that nothing can be done."

Studies have also pointed to the role of antioxidants in delaying the onset of crippling Alzheimer's disease. New evidence is showing that cholesterol in the arteries is linked to the creation of the plaques associated with Alzheimer's disease in the brain.

Researchers have found increased levels of fats in the nerve-cell linings of Alzheimer's sufferers, especially in the areas of the brain which control memory and attention functions.

The brain cells were more resilient when scientists were able to block the accumulation of these fats through dietary restrictions.

"At the very least, maintaining a lifestyle that reduces heart disease might also lower your risk of getting demented," said Dr. Wolozin.

In a study of rats, researchers from the National Institute on Aging reported recently that fasting every other day triggered an increase in the normal growth of new brain cells. The regimen also increased the production of needed substances, such as heat-shock protein-70, which helps prevent damage to brain cells. The study found that long intervals between meals seems to have a beneficial effect on brain cells, even if the overall number of calories eaten per day are not reduced.

Dr. Wolozin said researchers have found that cholesterol is a major source of the plaques that develop in the brain and which can ultimately cause Alzheimer's.

"The enzymes that produce plaques live in cholesterol and they need it to function," he said.

Antioxidants, too, have been found to be very beneficial in guarding brain cells from decay. One study done by the Institute for Brain Aging and Dementia at the University of California, Irvine, found that beagles fed vitamins C and E, as well as the supplements acetylcarnitine and alphalipoic acid, did better in memory tests than untreated dogs. Some older dogs, it was found, even got better.

Carl Cotman, director of the Institute and the leader of the study, said the antioxidant-rich diet reduced the amount of plaques in the brain of the treated dogs. "This is a tantalizing prospect for elderly humans," one account of the study said, "for whom mild cognitive decline is often seen as a normal sign of aging."

Other lifestyle choices you make can help your mental health and overall health.

One study found that people who stayed at their jobs until age 70 lived a year-and-a-half longer, on average, than those who retired at age 60.

Scientists are still analyzing the data, but it's safe to surmise that the people who worked at their careers longer also utilized their brains more. And, as noted above, it's beginning to look as if brains need workouts and exercise just as limbs and cardio-vascular systems do.

Science, in fact, is finding that intellectual pursuits are tied to overall well-being. And the saying "use it or lose it" is found to apply to the brain as well as other parts of the body.

In one recent study, researchers found that the risk of developing Alzheimer's disease is nearly four times greater in less-active people ages 20 to 60 than it is in more active people. "This seemed to be true regardless of the type of activity, although spending time in intellectual pursuits appeared to be most beneficial," the study noted.

"A passive life is not best for the brain," said the study. "The brain is an organ just like every other organ of the body. Just as physical activity is good for the heart, muscles and lungs, learning is important for keeping the brain healthy."

Traveling, learning a musical instrument or learning a foreign language can challenge and stimulate the brain.

The researchers asked study participants about their leisure activities and found that physical activities were most likely to be sports, working out in a gym, riding a bicycle, gardening, ice skating and jogging. Intellectual activities included reading, doing puzzles, playing a musical instrument, painting, woodworking, playing cards and board games, and doing home repairs. Passive activities were watching TV, listening to music, talking on the telephone, visiting friends and attending church.

"People who participated in fewer activities than the average were 3.85 times more likely to develop the memory-robbing illness" of Alzheimer's, the study found.

"People with Alzheimer's disease were less

active in passive, physical and intellectual activities. Since intellectual activities appear to keep the brain healthy, adults should have more opportunities to participate in learning activities ... This is especially true for older people, who often are limited in what sort of activities they can participate in.

"Unfortunately," it was noted, "many elderly — and younger people as well — spend much of their leisure time watching television. The only activity that Alzheimer's patients performed more frequently than the healthy controls was watching television."

Scientists are finding that our brains seem to go into serious decline only if we allow them to by becoming intellectually inactive. One study found that elderly people who sing, paint or otherwise participate in the creation of some form of art are less likely to suffer from depression, make three fewer visits to the doctor each year and take fewer medications as well.

Stay social, stay active, eat right, exercise — they're turning out to be the main components in keeping mind and body healthy after age 40.

CHAPTER 18

Doctor, My Eyes

One of these mornings you who are in your early- to mid-40s are going to realize your local newspaper editors are playing tricks on you. The print in your local Picayune/Traveler/Gossipmonger may appear fuzzy and blurred. You may find yourself playing trombone in an attempt to pick out the small type — holding it waaaay out here at arm's length first, then bringing it waaay back in toward your nose. Do not, in your ire, write a scathing letter to said editors. For you have a very common, though dire sounding, condition known as presbyopia.

And presbyopia — a bending of the lenses of your eye that makes it difficult to see close objects — can be the least of your troubles when it comes to aging and your eyes. Reading glasses prescribed by your eye doctor can pretty much take care of presbyopia — but other vision problems that come with age can be much more serious.

One such problem, known as low vision, can affect some people as they age. "Low vision means you cannot fix your eyesight with glasses, contact lenses, medicine or surgery," notes the National Institute on Aging. "It can get in the way of your normal daily routine."

The NIA lists the following symptoms of low vision:

- **Trouble seeing well enough to do everyday tasks like cooking, reading or sewing**
- **Trouble recognizing the faces of friends and family**
- **Trouble reading street signs**

● **A sensation that lights aren't as bright as usual**

If you have any or all of the above symptoms, ask your eye doctor to test you for low vision. If you do in fact have it, don't despair. "There are many things that can help," says the NIA. "Aids can help you read, write and manage daily living tasks. Lighting can be adjusted to your needs. You can also try prescription reading glasses, large-print materials, magnifying aids, closed-circuit televisions, audio tapes, electronic reading machines and computers that use large print and speech."

Experts recommend that people have a regular eye examination at least every two years. "The eye-care professional should check your eyesight, your glasses and your eye muscles," says the NIA.

Besides the nuisance of presbyopia and the more dire problem of low vision, your eye-care professional can also check for the following eye problems that are common with age — but which can "lead to vision loss and blindness" if left untreated, notes the NIA:

● **Dry eye.** This condition occurs when the tear glands stop working well. The condition can cause itching, burning and some loss of vision. Correcting the problem could involve eye drops or a home humidifier to prevent your eyes from drying out — but the remedy could also involve surgery.

● **Glaucoma.** The buildup of fluid pressure inside the eye is known as glaucoma. "Over time, the disease can damage the optic nerve," says the NIA. "This leads to vision loss and blindness. Loss of vision doesn't happen until there has been a large amount of nerve damage. Most people with glaucoma have no early symptoms or pain from increased pressure." Indeed, The Glaucoma Foundation estimates that of the 3 million people with glaucoma in the United States, half don't even know they have it. Having regular eye exams in which your pupils are dilated and the pressure measured can lead to early diagnosis and treatment, which may involve eye drops, oral medicines or even surgery. Experts are finding that vigorous exercise can help prevent the disease or relieve its effects if you have it. "Regular exercise can lower your intraocular pressure, the most significant risk factor for glaucoma," says Dr. Robert Ritch, medical director for The Glaucoma Foundation. "Keeping your pressure down can be very therapeutic." However, Dr. Ritch says certain activities — some yoga positions, scuba diving and, yes, bungee jumping are not advised for glaucoma patients as they can raise the pressure in your eyes.

● **Age-related macular degeneration (AMD).** The retina, which helps provide clear central vision, can over time become ruined and affect common daily activities, such as driving or reading. The macula, which is the central and most sensitive portion of the retina, can break down and the ability to distinguish fine detail becomes impaired while peripheral vision is maintained. If the macular function breaks down entirely, simple tasks such as reading can become impossible. AMD can be treated with lasers to decrease further vision loss and there is some research suggesting that dietary supplements may reduce the risk of getting AMD. While the exact cause of AMD remains unknown, risk factors for AMD include smoking, farsightedness, light-colored eyes and a family history of the disorder.

● **Diabetic retinopathy.** Diabetic retinopathy is another retinal disorder and is a common complication, obviously, of diabetes. It occurs when small blood vessels in your eyes stop feeding the retina, causing a loss of vision. Laser surgery and a procedure known as vitrectomy may help. Experts advise regular health exams to diagnose diabetes early. "If you have diabetes, be sure to have an eye exam through dilated pupils every year," recommends the NIA.

● **Retinal detachment.** The inner and outer layers of the retina can become separated over time, causing changes in "floaters" — those tiny specks that seem to float across your eyes — or light flashes in your eye. If you notice such changes, see your eye-care professional immediately. Through surgery or laser treatment, the retina can often be reattached and all or some of your eyesight can be restored.

● **Cataracts.** Cataracts, a slow thickening of the eye lens, causes vision to become cloudy and keeps light from passing through the eyes, causing loss of eyesight. They can form slowly with no symptoms and, while some become small and don't change much over time, others can become very thick and ruin vision. Cataract surgery can help restore vision. Your eye-care professional can monitor changes to the lenses over time through regular checkups.

"Although the presence of a visual disorder might seem obvious, many people are unaware that they have one," notes the Johns Hopkins *Health After 50* newsletter. "Surveys performed by researchers at Johns Hopkins found that about one-third of people with eye disease were unaware of it and that more than one third of people ages 65 to 84 had not visited an eye doctor in the last year. Periodic visits to an eye-care specialist are needed to detect conditions (such as glaucoma) early enough to allow effective treatment.

"If treated early enough, the most common eye disorders — cataracts, glaucoma, age-related macular degeneration and diabetic retinopathy — can often be slowed or halted with drugs, surgery or both. In addition, treating vision problems can enhance quality of life by allowing the person to return to such daily activities as driving, grocery shopping, using public transportation and performing household tasks."

So see your eye-care professional on a regular basis. And don't hesitate to see your doctor if these other, but comparatively minor, complaints arise:

● **Tearing.** A sudden rush of tears from your

eyes can be caused by being sensitive to wind, light or even temperature changes, or it could be a sign that you have dry eye (see above), an infection or blocked tear duct. Protecting the eyes better by wearing sunglasses can relieve symptoms in some cases.

● **Corneal diseases and problems.** The cornea, the clear, dome-shaped "window" at the front of the eye, helps focus light into the eye. But disease, infection, injury, toxic substances and other things can harm the eye and cause redness, watery eyes, reduced vision, eye pain and perhaps a halo effect in your vision, says the NIA. Treatment may simply be a matter of changing your eyeglass prescription or using eye drops — but in more severe cases, corneal transplantation may be warranted.

● **Conjunctivitis.** Also known as pink eye, conjunctivitis is an inflammation of the tissue that lines the eyelid and covers the cornea and may be caused by allergies or by an infection. Itching, burning, tearing or a feeling that an object is in your eye are common symptoms of conjunctivitis. While an infection causing the trouble can be easily spread to others, it also is easily treated.

CHAPTER 19

Take It Easy

Lighten up, while you still can — wasn't that the way the Eagles sang it way back in 1972?

Nah — it couldn't have been that long ago.

In the 30-plus years since that song hit the airwaves, taking it easy has become harder and harder. The stresses of everyday life — work, kids, money — have made us a nation of workaholics, as most families find it takes two wage-earners to provide our daily bread.

But stress can overload all of our systems and lay to waste our overall health.

"Recognize that stress is a killer," notes one writer. "A life filled with stress can really wreak havoc on your body, causing a number of illnesses such as heart attacks, strokes, asthma, gastric problems, menstrual disorders, ulcerative colitis, angina, increased blood pressure, ulcers, headaches, etc."

Stress is a part of life — and the question becomes how we deal with it. "All stress is not bad," notes one writer. "In fact, life would not be very interesting if it were not met with challenges. However, too much stress, too often with no effective and appropriate outlet, does not allow the body and soul to recuperate."

And don't worry so much or use denial and avoidance as a way to deal with problems. "Many worriers try to cope by not thinking about their problems, but this just makes things worse," the writer notes.

What is an "effective and appropriate" outlet? Getting smashed isn't. Nor are chain-smoking or resorting to binge eating. One of the best things you can do is exercise — work that stress off through vigorous physical activity.

Yoga and meditation are great ways to take a mental vacation from the stresses of your life as well. And, as noted before, make sure you are eating right. The combination of stress and poor nutrition can cut short your life.

And take regular vacations. One nine-year study of 12,000 males found that taking a vacation actually extended their lives. The study found that men who took an annual vacation were less likely to die from heart disease than were men who didn't give themselves a break.

And drink green tea (see previous chapter). Not only does the stuff lower blood pressure, prevent cancers and have all sorts of other wonderful healthy benefits, but it's been linked to stress reduction as well.

But before you get too relaxed, know this: One study says a little stress in our lives can actually promote health!

"Sustained stress definitely is not good for you," said Richard Morimoto, John Evans Professor of Biology at Northwestern, who co-authored the report *Molecular Biology of the Cell.* "But it appears that an occasional burst of stress or low levels of stress can be protective.

"Brief exposure to environmental and physiological stress has long-term benefits to the cell because it unleashes a great number of molecular chaperones that capture all kinds of damaged and misfolded proteins" — misformed proteins within a cell that, if left to accumulate, can develop into such neurodegenerative diseases as Huntington's, Parkinson's, Alzheimer's and Lou Gehrig's disease.

So a little stress is good.

Who knew the boss was right?

So shock yourself once in awhile. It could save your life!

Hand-in-hand with managing or even reducing the stress in your life is sleep.

How much sleep should you get? It may vary from person to person, but experts generally say seven or eight hours a night is right.

"You should sleep as much as you need to feel awake, alert and attentive the next day," says Daniel Buysse, a University of Pittsburgh psychiatrist and the past president of the American Academy of Sleep Medicine.

Stressed-out and overworked Americans, in particular, are a source of concern. Many Americans sleep when and where they can get it and live much of their lives in a sleep-deprived state. And in developed countries in general, in the past 100 years the average night's sleep has plummeted from nine hours to seven-and-a-half hours.

Too little sleep can accelerate the aging process, studies have found — and "chronic sleep loss may speed the onset or increase the severity of age-related conditions such as Type 2 diabetes, high blood pressure, obesity and memory loss," says one study published in the British medical journal *The Lancet.*

Though noting that "people who trade sleep for work or play may get used to it and feel less fatigued," the researchers found that blood-sugar levels of the men in the study "took 40 percent longer to drop following a high-carbohydrate meal, compared with the sleep-recovery period."

Overall, the changes in the sleep-deprived men mimicked the effects of insulin resistance — a warning sign of Type 2 diabetes. What's more, the sleep-deprived men had higher nighttime concentrations of cortisol, which regulates blood sugar, and lower levels of a thyroid-stimulating hormone. "These raised cortisol levels mimic levels that are often seen in older people and may be involved in age-related insulin resistance and memory loss," the study noted.

The changes in blood sugar and hormones were reversed with regular sleep. "An adequate amount of sleep is as important as an adequate amount of exercise," the journal noted. "Sleeping is not a sin."

Older people often suffer from sleep troubles with an inability to sleep — insomnia — being the most common complaint. Also, a common disorder known as sleep apnea, of which there are two types, can rob the elderly of sleep.

Obstructive sleep apnea occurs when there is an involuntary pause in breathing and air cannot flow in or out of a person's nose or mouth. Central sleep apnea, which is less common, occurs when the brain doesn't send the right messages to the breathing muscles and breathing pauses.

This struggle to breathe all night can leave a person sleep-deprived. Sleep apnea is treatable, however, and can include learning to sleep in another position. Treatment can also include using devices that keep airways open and, in extreme cases, medications and surgery.

Treating insomnia or sleep apnea is extremely important. A study of 185 people ages 59 to 91 found that those who spent more than 30 minutes trying to fall asleep were more than twice as likely to die within 13 years as those who were able to fall asleep more quickly. People who slept less were almost twice as likely to die during the time frame of the study.

Quality of sleep also played a role in maintaining health. Those who got an average amount of REM — or dream phase sleep — lived longer than those who got the least amount, the study found.

Sleep troubles can also foreshadow the onset of other life-shortening afflictions. People with dementia and depression often undergo changes in the length and quality of their sleep first.

Experts give these tips for getting to sleep — and staying there:

● *Follow a regular sleep schedule* — go to bed and get up at the same time each day.

And try to limit napping during the day if you are having trouble falling asleep at night.

● *Don't drink alcohol or smoke cigarettes* in an effort to knock yourself out. Even small amounts of alcohol can make it harder to stay asleep and tobacco, a stimulant, can make it harder for you to fall asleep.

● *Exercise* each day to tire yourself out and induce sleep.

● *Don't drink beverages with caffeine* late in the day.

● *Create a safe and comfortable area* for sleeping. The room should be quiet, dark and well-ventilated.

● *Beware of hidden stimulants* such as chocolate or anything flavored with coffee, as well as herbal teas with guarana or ginseng.

● *Develop a routine* at night for going to bed and stick to it. For instance, taking a hot bath, reading a book or magazine or watching the news could be the last thing you do before bed each night.

● *Try not to focus on everyday worries* as you try to fall asleep. Worrying will only cause stress and keep you awake.

   Later. Gotta get some z's.

CHAPTER 20

Not Feelin' So Good Myself

Bye-bye. See ya later. Be well.

It sounds so easy.

But, of course, there are times when you're just plain old not going to be well, no matter how much you exercise or how well you eat.

Still, there are things you can do to at least minimize your likelihood of catching a bug like the flu, which each year strikes millions of Americans and which, in cases where immune systems have been compromised by age or general poor health, can lead to death or a further breakdown in health.

But vitamins, good nutrition, exercise and getting plenty of rest can help your body fight off the virus when you are exposed, as well as reduce your flu exposure in the first place.

Said Dr. Elliot Dick, MD, chief of the Respiratory Virus Research Laboratory and Professor of Preventive Medicine at the University of Wisconsin School of Medicine:

"There is nothing that anyone can do to completely protect themselves from coming down with the flu this winter because there are more than 150 different upper respiratory viruses out there that can give a person cold and flu symptoms.

"Flu shots only help build immunity to two of them — and at its best even then, it only gives you 50 percent protection against just those two viruses.

"But your immune system is involved in fighting all of the cold and flu viruses, so your best bet of beating colds and the flu is boosting your immune system in as many ways as possible to help it effectively ward off flu and cold viruses."

Said Dr. William Adler, MD, chief of clinical immunology at the National Institute on Aging: "By using key vitamins and eating a healthy diet, as well as getting plenty of rest and exercise, you can ensure that your immune system is in top shape to fight off the flu virus."

Top experts recommend the following to prevent or at least minimize the effects of the flu:

● **Take daily doses of the key immune-boosting vitamins C and E, and the trace mineral zinc.**

Said an expert: "One of the byproducts of normal metabolism is free radicals—microscopic substances that can be very damaging to your body's cells. Free radicals contribute to various disease processes and also reduce the effectiveness of your body's immune system.

"But other substances, called 'antioxidants,' help protect the body against damage caused by free radicals. Certain vitamins are themselves antioxidants and the body uses other vitamins to make enzymes that act as antioxidants.

"There is good evidence in both humans and animals that antioxidants can help prevent certain diseases and can help boost the effectiveness of the immune system in fighting infections."

● **Take 100-200 mg of vitamin E per day.**

Said one expert: "Vitamin E is a fat-soluble antioxidant that inhibits the formation of highly toxic free radicals in and around the cell membranes. It helps protect cells and the DNA they carry from repeated damage that may be one of the fundamental causes of aging.

"Animal studies have shown that it increases the immune response of mice, chickens, turkeys and sheep. And it has been shown to increase the survival of these animals when they are infected with bacteria or viruses," according to the studies.

"The amount of vitamin E we're recommending is over the 1-mg RDA — but it is nontoxic."

● **Take one to two grams of Vitamin C each day.**

Said Dr. Dick: "I studied the effectiveness of vitamin C against cold viruses in humans and I was turned from an absolute skeptic into someone who is a faithful vitamin C user.

"My study done here at the University of Wisconsin demonstrated that by taking 2 grams of vitamin C every day, people exposed to cold viruses avoided catching the colds, while those who were given placebo did get infected. Now I hardly ever get colds or flu — nor does my family."

● **Eat regular, healthy meals.**

Said Dr. Adler: "This is a key element in keeping your immune system functioning properly. Make sure you eat plenty of fruits and vegetables, particularly vitamin-C-rich citrus fruits and dark green leafy vegetables that are rich in beta-carotene. Also make sure your diet is relatively low in fat and high in fiber.

"Good nutrition is essential to a properly functioning immune system," added Dr. Dick. "I recommend a low-fat diet that contains plenty of fruits and vegetables and whole grains."

● **Exercise regularly — at least 30 minutes a day five days a week.**

Said Dr. Adler: "Regular exercise can definitely help people reduce their risk of viral infection. It helps keep the body's immune system functioning well and it also has very positive effects on the lungs and upper airways. It helps aerate the whole of the lung field, so there are no stagnant areas that can be a set up for infection."

"A half hour a day five days a week is a good amount to aim for," added Dr. Dick. "This can include anything from walking, bike riding or running to tennis, aerobics or calisthenics.

"But if you haven't been exercising, make sure you check with your physician before you start any program of regular exercise. And start slowly at first, say with walking for a few weeks before you move up to jogging."

● **Get plenty of rest during flu season.**

Dr. Adler said, "Getting rundown and low on sleep can be a set up for the flu. Getting enough rest is important to keep your immune system functioning well.

"I recommend at least seven hours of sleep each night. If this is a problem — and it is for many older people who just don't sleep that long at night — take naps."

● **Keep stress under control.**

"Many studies have shown that chronic

emotional stress can harm the immune system and lead to a variety of diseases," said Dr. Adler. "The problem is that what's stressful for one person may not be stressful for another.

"The key here is to know yourself. Learning to relax and relieve your stress through meditation, recreation, exercise or whatever works best for you can make a big difference in your health and help you avoid succumbing to various illnesses, including the flu."

● **Dress warmly for winter weather and avoid getting chilled.**

"Excessive exposure to cold weather can be a set up for various illness, especially in the elderly," said Dr. Adler. "Over time, it can reduce the efficiency of the immune system and make infections with cold and flu virus more likely. Mortality figures skyrocket in the elderly during the wintertime — and this is one of the major reasons why."

This is simply good common sense, but it's valid: Make sure when you go out in cold or damp weather to dress appropriately and limit your exposure.

● **If you are older than age 50 make sure to get a flu shot.**

"Flu can have its most serious and lethal effects on the elderly, so it is a good idea for anyone over age 50 to get a flu vaccination," said Dr. Adler.

● **Cover your nose and mouth when someone else coughs or sneezes near you and make sure family members stricken with flu use good basic hygiene.**

"It's easy to tell people to avoid crowds during flu season, but that's actually very hard to do," noted Dr. Adler. "Your life doesn't stop just because it's flu season.

"But colds and flu are primarily spread through tiny droplets in the air after people cough or sneeze. So when someone coughs or sneezes near you, turn your head, cover your nose and mouth and, if you can, leave the immediate area.

"Basic hygiene can play a very major role in preventing the flu and colds. The flu sufferer himself can do a lot to prevent the spread of the virus. The Japanese often wear little face masks to prevent the spread of cold and flu virus through aerosol droplets when they sneeze and cough — but that's not a custom in this country.

"However, if you make sure that anyone

in your family who has the flu uses disposable tissues, covers their mouth when they sneeze and cough and doesn't leave used dishes and glasses around that might be used by others — this will help reduce the spread of infection."

"Most colds and flu are transmitted through continuous contact with the infected person, as in a home," said Dr. Dick. If somebody in your house has a cold or the flu you are likely to catch it — about 50 to 60 percent. In this case, the individual who has the cold should be careful to cover their nose and mouth when they cough or sneeze and blow their nose into tissues that can be discarded rather than into a handkerchief, which becomes a haven for germs. Every time you yank it out of your pocket it spreads the virus around.

"But in public, it's fairly difficult to catch a cold in a short period of time — one or two hours — unless you're unlucky. There's one exception — if you hear someone really coughing away. That's the time to move in the other direction."

● **Avoid dry atmospheres and use a humidifier at home.**

"A lot of people have forced air heating and

this can cause a very dry atmosphere in the winter," said Dr. Adler. "This has a negative effect on people's upper respiratory systems, drying out the epithelial tissues and actually helping cold and flu viruses gain entry.

"One of the reasons scientists think there is a much higher incidence of upper respiratory infection in the wintertime is because people spend so much more time in dry unhumidified air," said Dr. Dick. "We think this excessive dryness may keep the tiny cilia in our upper airways from moving to help rid us effectively of bacteria and viruses. If you humidify your home or workplace, you can partially avoid this problem."

You can also reduce the effects of an illness caused by the flu by taking flu-fighters such as Tamiflu or an inhaled powder called Relenza.

"These are real breakthroughs," said Dr. Frederick G. Hayden, MD, a professor of medicine at the University of Virginia School of Medicine. "When used early, they can reduce the duration and severity of the illness, get people back on their feet more quickly and reduce the risk of complications."

The experts say the drugs can work

against both Type A and Type B flu viruses, whereas older flu medications, amantadine and rimantadine, are effective only against Type A. They also can shorten the duration of flu bouts by up to two-and-a-half days and cause very few side effects, compared to the older drugs.

They also reduce complications from flu, including pneumonia and heart problems, by up to 50 percent. This is particularly important since flu hospitalizes about 300,000 Americans every year and kills 20,000 to 40,000.

Not only do the new drugs treat the flu, but recent studies show it actually can prevent the onset of symptoms among people who have been exposed to the virus.

Dr. Hayden and colleagues reported on two studies involving 1,559 patients. A third of those got 75 mg of Tamiflu once a day, a third got it twice a day and a third got placebo for six weeks during a peak flu period, he reports. The protective effectiveness of the drug was 82 percent, he says, and those in the placebo group developed the flu at twice the rate of either of the drug groups.

Studies show Relenza (zanamivir), a

powder spray inhaled through the mouth, also cuts the risk of flu by nearly 80 percent for those just exposed.

In one study of 975 families in which 337 had a family member with the flu, either Relenza or a look-alike placebo was given. The result: Only 4 percent of those getting the drug came down with the flu, compared to 19 percent of those who got the placebo. What's more, Dr. Hayden reports, those who did get sick got over the flu faster and had much less severe symptoms.

"There will never be a more cost-effective way to protect against influenza than vaccine, but if the vaccine doesn't work because the virus has changed, these drugs will do the job," Dr. Hayden said. "And when the next worldwide epidemic occurs, they could make an enormous difference. People now need to understand if they develop influenza, there are treatments available; it's no longer necessary to stay home and hope the misery will go away.

"The treatments are best when they are given very early. People usually know when they've been hit by flu because it's not a subtle illness; it hits hard with fever, chills, aches and pains — misery. That's when people should seek treatment with these drugs."

You should watch for chills, fever ranging from 101 to 103, sore throat, runny nose, muscle aches, headaches, extreme fatigue, a dry cough, chills, diarrhea and dizziness. The most common of these are fever, coughs and muscle aches; the others also could signal a cold. Flu symptoms come on quickly and are more severe than the same symptoms with a cold.

So if you thought there was nothing you could do to prevent you or your family members from getting the flu, think again. Be proactive, stay on top of your health and the health of your loved ones.

Oh, yes — and eat your vegetables.

CHAPTER 21

Gummin' the Works

Open up.

Hmmph.

No, wider.

Umph-mph.

That's it. Hold it right there. So, how ya been?

Hmmmmppmphnn.

Don't worry. We'll do the talking.

We want to talk about your mouth. We're not horse-traders, just concerned citizens. And we want to make sure that when it comes to your health, you're not neglecting one of the places good health begins — the mouth.

It's hard to eat without teeth, but many people allow their teeth and gums to slip way, way down the depth chart when thinking about their overall health. But gum disease, the product of neglected oral health, can not only lead to more serious troubles such as heart disease. New research is finding that the presence of gum disease can signal more serious problems with your health.

"It wasn't too long ago that inflammation below the gum line, often accompanied by bad breath and occasional bleeding, was considered a not-too-serious, easily treated infection," says one account. "But new studies show that gum disease — gingivitis and periodontitis — can be symptomatic of many ailments. It is even linked to bringing on preterm labor in pregnant women."

"Not only does destruction caused by periodontitis take away a person's ability to speak, eat and smile with comfort and confidence, the mounting evidence suggests that it also contributes to heart disease, the risk of premature, underweight births — and poses a serious threat to people whose health is already compromised by diabetes and respiratory diseases," said Dr. Michael Rethman, president of the American Academy of Periodontology.

The warning symptoms of gum disease include:

- *Loose teeth*
- *A change in the way your teeth fit together when you bite*
- *A change in the fit of partial dentures*
- *Bleeding gums when you brush or floss*
- *Red, swollen or tender gums*
- *Bad breath that won't go away no matter what you try*
- *Gums that have pulled away from your teeth*
- *Dry mouth*
- *Teeth grinding (which can cause cracked or chipped teeth and can increase the risk of developing periodontal disease)*
- *Genetics (a large segment of the population may be susceptible to developing severe periodontal diseases, but early testing can help identify and treat at-risk patients)*

But there are simple ways to prevent gum

disease. "The good news is that it's totally treatable," said Dr. Sally Cram, a consumer advisor for the American Dental Association.

In its early stages, gingivitis can usually be reversed with careful cleaning of the gums. But if left untreated, it can develop into the more serious and stubborn periodontitis, which leads to bacteria that can spread from the mouth to other parts of the body and set up an infection, said Dr. Cram.

To prevent gum disease, experts advise that you make regular visits — at least twice yearly — to a dentist. A thorough cleaning is essential to prevent periodontal disease.

Experts also advise you to:

- **Brush your teeth well at least twice a day.** Use a soft-bristled toothbrush and use toothpastes and mouth rinses that contain fluoride.

- **Clean your teeth every day.** Use a floss or interdental cleaner to remove bacteria and food particles your toothbrush can't reach.

- **Clean under the gum** collar around the base of your teeth.

- **Eat a balanced diet.**

- **Quit smoking.** Smoking dramatically increases the chance of periodontal disease and/or oral cancer.
- **Have tartar removed.** Your dentist or oral hygienist can remove the calcified plaque in places where your toothbrush and floss can't reach.

And remember — bad health bites.

CHAPTER 22

It's a Drinkin' Thing

And what about a drink? A snort? A belt? A little pick-me-up?

We're happy to answer that alcohol in moderation is, in fact, becoming recognized for its role in promoting health.

Scientists began noticing several decades ago that as much as the French smoked, ate fatty foods and drank wine, they had low rates of cardiovascular and other diseases. The observations became known as the French paradox.

Some investigation brought out the fact that wine, and especially the French reds, seemed to be the source of all that robust health. Further investigation into the benefits of red wine — and alcohol in general — has continued to bring more and more evidence that drinking, in moderation, can ward off a variety of ills and help us remain healthy.

One recent study reported that having two drinks a day can cut the risk of a heart attack by 25 percent. "It's about the same risk reduction for heart attack that a person who was overweight by 30 pounds would achieve by losing 30 pounds," said Eric Rimm, associate professor of epidemiology and nutrition at the Harvard School of Public Health.

The study found that having more than two drinks per day gave even greater cardiovascular benefits — but experts remain wary of recommending more than two drinks per day, even for men, because of elevated risks for other health problems, such as cancers, high blood pressure, alcoholism and bleeding disorders.

The Harvard scientists said in the report that alcohol in moderate amounts increased the level of HDL, or good, cholesterol and also reduced clotting in blood, which can be a factor in artery blockages.

However, the scientists did not recommend that people who had been teetotallers begin drinking for "medicinal purposes." But "for those who drink moderately, this new evidence suggests they are reducing their risk of heart attack by about a quarter," said Rimm.

Moderate drinking has also been found to significantly reduce the risk of stroke. The study, published in the *New England Journal of Medicine*, tracked 22,000 men for an average of 12 years each and found that even one drink a week could cut the chance of ischemic strokes — those caused by blockage of a blood vessel — by 20 percent compared with nondrinkers.

Though the study focused on men, study co-author Dr. Julie Buring, professor of preventative medicine at Brigham and Women's Hospital, said she couldn't identify "any physiological reason" alcohol wouldn't work the same way on women.

However, it was noted that drinking heavily — five or more drinks per day — significantly raises the risk of stroke. "There's a fine line between the beneficial and the harmful," Dr. Buring said.

There's more promising news related to alcohol and health. A recent study found that light to moderate amounts of alcohol may help prevent degenerative diseases such as Alzheimer's and other types of dementia in people older than age 65.

A study published in 2003 in the *Journal of the American Medical Association* involved 373 elderly people with dementia and 373 elderly people who were fit. "Abstainers had odds of dementia that were about twice as high as the odds among consumers of between one and six drinks per week," the report said. Heavier drinkers, those who were considered moderate and had between seven and 14 drinks per week, had the same lowered risks of dementia.

Light drinkers had a 54 percent less chance of developing dementia as did those who abstained from drinking alcohol, the study found. Moderate drinkers had a 31 percent lower chance — but heavy drinkers were 22 percent more likely to develop dementia than were those who didn't drink.

The type of alcoholic drink — beer, wine, spirits — didn't matter, according to the study.

If you don't drink, hold that thought. There's no reason to rush to the bar and begin pounding them down now.

But if you like a drink, maybe even one or two a day, go ahead and belly up to the bar. It won't hurt you as much as they used to say — and may possibly help your health more than we even know.

Research into another socially stigmatized area of imbibing is also turning up good news when it comes to staying healthy.

Though you're the odd duck in this country if you drink tea, the fact is, whether it's green or black, tea is being found to have great health benefits.

The Japanese and Chinese have long known about the health-giving benefits of tea, especially green tea — and Western scientists are finally catching up with those claims and are finding that teas do, indeed, measure up.

Tea, research is finding, can help reduce your risks of heart disease, cancer, kidney stones, osteoporosis and even gum disease.

Here's a summary of the latest research on the health benefits of tea:

● **Heart Disease.** In a study published in the *Journal of Nutrition,* USDA researchers found that people who drank five cups of black tea each day for three weeks saw their levels of LDL cholesterol — the "bad" cholesterol — decrease by an amazing 11 percent, with an average decline of 7.5 percent.

Another study at Brigham and Women's Hospital and Harvard Medical School examined 340 men and women who had suffered heart attacks and found that those who drank a cup or more of black tea daily reduced their heart attack risk by an incredible 44 percent.

And a 1999 study of 3,454 men and women in the Netherlands found that drinking two cups of black tea daily reduced the risk of aortic atherosclerosis — hardening of the arteries — by an amazing 69 percent!

● **Cancer.** Japanese researchers surveyed 8,552 people over age 40 for nine years and found that women who drank 10 or more cups of green tea daily had an astonishing

43 percent lower cancer risk than women who drank fewer than three cups. For men the risk was 32 percent lower.

Another study, "The Iowa Women's Study," followed postmenopausal women between ages 55 and 69 for eight years. It found that those women who drank two or more cups of tea daily had a 32 percent lower risk of developing digestive tract cancers and a 60 percent lower risk of developing urinary tract cancers.

And at the 2001 Congress of Epidemiology in Toronto, researchers from Moscow reported finding that women who were regular tea drinkers had a much lower risk of rectal cancer than women who aren't.

● **Kidney stones.** A five-year study of 81,000 women found that regular tea drinkers had a lower risk of developing kidney stones.

● **Osteoporosis.** A recent study in the *American Journal of Clinical Nutrition* reported that older women who drank tea had a higher bone mineral density than those who didn't drink tea.

● **Oral health.** A study at the University of Illinois/Chicago found that people who rinsed their mouths with black tea reduced the amount of decay-causing plaque that formed on their teeth.

Further, scientists at the Beltsville Human Nutrition Research Center in Beltsville, Maryland, studied the effect of tea on the metabolism of fats and found that people who drank five cups of tea daily burned 12 percent more fat calories than those who drank water.

Scientists credit the polyphenols in green tea, elements of the plant which contain certain antioxidants — which, as we know, are important in quelling disease-promoting free radicals.

"Researchers from around the world, from Hong Kong to the Netherlands, have shown that green tea lowers blood pressure, blood cholesterol and helps prevent atherosclerosis," notes an article in a recent *Macrobiotics Today*. "It has also been reported that elements in green tea prolong the life span in stroke-prone individuals, protect against genetic mutations and are effective against a wide variety of cancers."

The American Heart Association reported in a study that drinking green tea could help lower the chances that a victim of a heart attack would die following the attack. Heavy tea drinkers — those who drink two or more cups per day — had a 44 percent lower death rate following a heart attack. The reason? Antioxidants in the tea seem to protect the heart by relaxing blood vessels.

Scientists at Case Western Reserve University studied the elements of green tea and found that one chemical in the tea, called EGCg, helped alleviate the effects of sunburn when applied topically. The substance is also credited for reducing metabolic changes in skin that can lead to skin cancer. "It has been shown," noted one publication, "that green tea applied to the skin as well as ingested can significantly reduce the formation of wrinkles."

More research from Case Western Reserve found that the antioxidants in green tea may prevent the onset of collagen-induced arthritis — arthritis which is caused by autoimmune diseases, such as rheumatoid arthritis and systemic lupus erythematosis.

Drinking green tea has also been linked to a reduction in the incidence of breast cancer in women. One study found that women who drank half a cup a day of green tea had a 47 percent reduced risk of breast cancer compared to those who did not drink the stuff.

Another study found that men who drank three cups of green tea per day had just a quarter of the risk of developing prostate cancer as did, uh, "green teetotallers."

And green tea also seems to benefit the cardiovascular system. A study published in the *Journal of Nutrition* in 2003 associated drinking green tea with lower blood pressure. Green tea has also been linked to a lower incidence of stroke and heart disease. Black tea, as noted above, has health-giving benefits — but it's made by fermenting green tea and the process dilutes some of the beneficial compounds. Noted one writer: "While studies show that black tea has the potential to benefit health, the research suggests that it's green tea that deserves the cup."

CHAPTER 23

Do You Believe in Magic?

Say, Mr. Wizard, beyond exercise and diet, is there a way to find therapies and potions that turn back our body clocks and reverse the effects of aging? You know, something that comes in a handy little pill?

Well, Timmy, we didn't want to go into this, but the answer is ...

No.

Not yet, anyway.

We only bring this up because in the past dozen years or more, there has been something of a frenzy regarding so-called "miracle" cures for aging, especially hormonal treatments. But the proof behind these remedies is fuzzy at best and there's no evidence that anything short of serious sweat, a balanced diet and some self-discipline at the dinner table are the reigning miracles when it comes to maintaining health after age 40.

Two hormonal treatments, in particular, have become mini-growth industries on their own, even as serious science tries to catch up and determine their true effects on the human body.

One, known as HGH, is secreted by the pituitary gland and is key to growth in children. It also helps the body turn fat into energy and keeps tissues and organs healthy into adulthood. "This process is essential in childhood and adolescence," notes the Mayo Clinic. "Without it, children remain short and become fat. But with

HGH therapy, these children usually grow taller and thinner."

The consideration of HGH (which the body produces in much smaller quantities as we age) as a device to turn back our bodies' clocks stems from research done in Wisconsin in 1990, when it was reported that 12 older men who had received shots of HGH three times a week over six months had become lean and muscular. Their bones, it was reported, also were strengthened by the therapy and their skin became tougher while their body fat decreased.

"The effects of six months of human growth hormone on lean body mass and adipose-tissue mass were equivalent in magnitude to the changes incurred during 10 to 20 years of aging," the Medical College of Wisconsin reported. The study created a sensation in anti-aging circles — and also set off a rush to apply HGH as an everyday tool to reverse the effects of aging and extend human life.

Since then, clinics and companies offering human growth hormones have sprung up, "many promising that their products — usually ineffective powders, pills or liquids that are sniffed or taken by mouth — will boost your levels of growth hormone and help you turn back your biological clock," says the Mayo Clinic.

"Middle-age baby boomers undeterred by hefty monthly price tags are turning to growth hormone shots to halt time — even as their effectiveness and safety remain unproven," says the Mayo Clinic. "Their eagerness to slow the inevitable and keep their competitive edge has spawned an industry and sparked a debate pitting the medical establishment against maverick physicians willing to prescribe regular, perhaps daily, injections to ward off the body's decline."

Indeed, the Anti-Aging Group, on its AAG Health Web site, claims that HGH therapy has been shown to benefit skin elasticity, provide more energy, improve bone strength and muscle mass, and also improve mental functioning, among other things.

"There have always been things you can do to 'stay young.' You can be born with good genes, eat healthy foods, exercise regularly, watch your weight, avoid stress and get enough quality sleep," the site says. "As good as these practices are, they can only delay and postpone the signs, symptoms and problems of aging. For years, researchers have hunted for a more dramatic key to staying young. Now, after centuries of seeking the 'Fountain of Youth,' it appears that medical science has achieved the first major breakthrough: human growth hormone therapy."

While the claims continue to be investigated by the federal government, "The only approved use for HGH is a shot given to children whose bodies do not make enough growth hormone," says the National Institute on Aging. "Only doctors may prescribe and give HGH shots. Despite this, some people spend thousands of dollars a year on these shots because they hope to slow down their bodies' aging. Others, who cannot afford the injections, buy over-the-counter 'HGH releasers.' Claims that these releasers will make the body 'release' more HGH are unproven."

In fact, further research has resulted in contradictory information on the effects of growth hormone. Mice bred to overproduce growth hormone died of malignant tumors, and at a younger age, than mice with lowered levels of growth hormone. Decreased levels of growth hormones in lab animals, in fact, seems to lead to increased life expectancy.

"What scientists do know is that in recent studies, injections of growth hormone for a short time seemed to boost the size and strength of muscles and to lessen body fat in a small group of older men and women," says the National Institutes of Health. "Longer studies with larger numbers of older people are needed to find out if HGH can prevent weakness and frailty in older people without causing dangerous side effects."

DHEA has also been touted as a "miracle" anti-aging hormone. It, too, is controversial — some studies have shown that DHEA builds muscle, but other studies have not shown the same effect. "When given to mice," reports the National Institute on Aging, "it boosted some components of the immune system and helped prevent some kinds of cancer."

As with HGH, levels of DHEA are naturally high in younger people and decrease with age. Our bodies turn DHEA into two sex hormones — testosterone and estrogen; in some people, DHEA can promote the production of large amounts of both of these hormones, which "could be dangerous," notes the NIA.

"High levels of naturally made testosterone in men and estrogen in women may play a role in prostate cancer in men and breast cancer in women. Experts do not know if supplements of DHEA will increase your chance of developing these cancers.

"Some people hope DHEA will improve energy and immunity, increase muscles and decrease body fat, but there is not enough research to support these claims or even to show taking DHEA is safe."

In other words, while DHEA, like human growth hormone, shows some early promise as a means to increase strength in older people, once again much more investigation into DHEA's side effects and long-term effects needs to be performed. And the National Institute on Aging warns people away from DHEA. "Scientists," the NIA says, "are somewhat mystified by DHEA and have not fully sorted out what it does in the body.

"Researchers are working to find more

definite answers about DHEA's effects on aging, muscles and the immune system," says the NIA. "In the meantime, people who are thinking about taking supplements of this hormone should understand that its effects are not fully known. Some of these unknown effects might turn out to be harmful."

The bottom line is this: Don't believe everything you read about these "miracle" hormones. Always talk to your doctor before taking any kind of medication or therapy.

Another hormone, melatonin, can be bought as a supplement. It is pushed in this form as a sleep aid, an anti-aging remedy and as a powerful antioxidant — and early studies have indicated that melatonin may indeed be effective against free radicals in large doses. But "claims that melatonin can slow or reverse aging are very far from proven," says the NIA.

Can testosterone have an effect upon age-related frailty, as some claim? As with HGH, DHEA and melatonin, the answer is currently unknown. Preliminary studies have been inconclusive. Also unknown is whether men who do not produce much testosterone later in life would derive any benefit from taking supplements. As mentioned above, there is some concern that testosterone supplements can increase the risk of prostate cancer — the second-leading cause of cancer death among men.

"For those few men who have extreme testosterone deficiencies, supplements in the form of patches, injections or a topical gel may offer substantial benefit," says the NIA. "Supplements may help a man with exceptionally low testosterone levels maintain strong muscles and bones, and increase sex drive. However, what effects testosterone replacement may have in healthy older men without these extreme deficiencies requires more research."

Finis

We're going to end by quoting one of our favorite philosophers, a woman of endless and deep insight, a woman who has never blanched from tackling the existential issues of our time head-on. Yeah, a woman who through deed and spoken word has become one of our most revered cultural icons ...

Of course, we're talking about ... Cher.

Well, it was Cher who once said *If I could turn back ti-uuum.* No, it was something else. Something in one of those TV commercials of hers to the effect of if great bodies came in a bottle, everyone would have one.

Segue, if you please. Yes, if good health after 40 could be achieved from a pill or a bottle, we'd all be walking around today in toned, youthful bodies with nary a hint of inner arterial-wall plaques, menacing polyps or fatty buildups in our livers.

But the ability to *Never Get Sick* doesn't come in a bottle or pill. Health, as we have seen, class, is the result of:

- A balanced diet chock-full of vitamins and minerals.
- Careful medical screening and testing.
- A proactive interest in our bodies.
- Vigorous exercise.
- Not smoking and not drinking to excess.
- More exercise.
- Getting enough rest.

In sum, learning to *Never Get Sick* means taking care of yourself — and helping others, ie., your health-care professional, help you take care of yourself. It means having a little self-discipline, laying off the junk food and not letting problems develop through behavior or neglect to the point where medical catastrophe looms.

Be good to yourself, be smart.

Never Get Sick.

Index

Order These Great Health & Fitness Books:

Please send the books checked below:

	Price Ea.	Qty.	Total
☐ **Instant Weight Loss** — Lose 10 pounds in 10 days — and keep it off!	$5.99		
☐ **No More Diets . ... Ever** — The breakthrough plan that will change your life	$5.99		
☐ **The Ultimate Low-Carb Plan** — The last diet book you'll ever buy	$5.99		
☐ **Instant Family Fitness** — A parent's guide to keeping your family healthy & happy	$5.99		
☐ **Change Your Luck** — The scientific way to improve your life!	$6.99		
☐ **Live :Longer, Look Younger** — Scientific breakthroughs you can use now	$5.99		

Postage & Handling:
U.S., $ 2.75 for one book, $ 1.00 for each additional

Total enclosed:

Ship to:

NAME _____

ADDRESS _____

CITY _____ STATE _____ ZIP _____

Please make your check or money order payable to AMI Books and mail it along with this order form to AMI Mail Order Books, 1000 American Media Way, Boca Raton, FL 33464-1000. Allow 4-6 weeks for delivery. Payable in U.S. funds only. No cash or COD accepted. We accept check or money orders ($15.00 fee for returned check). **Offer not available in Canada.**

0205SHAF